Débora D`Agostini Jorge Lisboa
Eliane Lucia Colussi
Marlene Doring

Anxiety, depression and heart surgery

Débora D`Agostini Jorge Lisboa
Eliane Lucia Colussi
Marlene Doring

Anxiety, depression and heart surgery

The relationship between anxiety and depression and pre- and post-cardiac surgery

ScienciaScripts

Imprint
Any brand names and product names mentioned in this book are subject to trademark, brand or patent protection and are trademarks or registered trademarks of their respective holders. The use of brand names, product names, common names, trade names, product descriptions etc. even without a particular marking in this work is in no way to be construed to mean that such names may be regarded as unrestricted in respect of trademark and brand protection legislation and could thus be used by anyone.

Cover image: www.ingimage.com

This book is a translation from the original published under ISBN 978-3-330-76856-7.

Publisher:
Sciencia Scripts
is a trademark of
Dodo Books Indian Ocean Ltd. and OmniScriptum S.R.L publishing group

120 High Road, East Finchley, London, N2 9ED, United Kingdom
Str. Armeneasca 28/1, office 1, Chisinau MD-2012, Republic of Moldova, Europe
Managing Directors: Ieva Konstantinova, Victoria Ursu
info@omniscriptum.com

Printed at: see last page
ISBN: 978-620-8-60010-5

SUMMARY

DEDICATORY

"As we come to the end of this work, we think how wonderful it is to do what we love. During our journey, we always come up against obstacles, sometimes difficult, sometimes easy, and we are forced to face them head on."

I dedicate this work to God for guiding and enlightening my life.

To my parents, Nei and Marlene, for life, for their example, encouragement, love and affection.

To my husband, Renato, for his encouragement, example, support, affection and patience. For being by my side at every stage of my life, sharing the best moments.

ACKNOWLEDGMENTS

I would like to thank my dear advisors and co-supervisors, Eliane Colussi and Marlene Doring, for their encouragement, patience, teaching and enthusiasm and, above all, for the affection they shared.

To the scholarship students, Gabriela and Luana, for their dedication, effort and commitment. For taking part alongside me on this long journey.

To the residents, Jûlia and Isadora, for their help and dedication.

To my colleague Indaiara, who was always there when I needed her most, for her cooperation, partnership and complicity.

To my colleague and friend Gabriela Mendonça, who has been with me throughout this journey, always a partner and faithful to our friendship. Whenever I needed it, she encouraged me and helped me to successfully complete this stage.

To my husband Renato, for being by my side at all the most important moments in my life, always encouraging me to seek new horizons. For his companionship, complicity, support and patience during this long and tortuous journey. You are part of this achievement!

To my parents, Nei and Marlene, for their lifelong teaching. For always being there for me at all times.

To my uncle and godfather Rudah Jorge, for his hospitality, dedication and teaching. For helping and accompanying this project from start to finish by my side;

To the secretary of the Postgraduate Program in Human Ageing, Rita, for her help and affection.

To the City and Sao Vicente de Paulo Hospitals, for opening their doors with great affection and allowing this research to be carried out.

To the patients, for making it possible for this study to happen, and for turning it from a dream into a reality. Thank you all from the bottom of my heart for everything.

Finally, to God, for allowing all this to happen with wisdom. For allowing long processes to be transformed into personal and professional growth.

EPILOGUE

"Every dream you leave behind is a piece of your future that no longer exists."

Steve Jobs

"There are no impossible dreams for those who truly believe that the fulfilling power resides within every human being, whenever someone discovers this power something previously considered impossible becomes a reality."

Albert Einstein

SUMMARY

Chronic heart disease is a highly prevalent group of pathologies worldwide, especially related to the phenomenon of population aging observed in recent years. Among the therapeutic modalities available for these diseases is cardiac surgery, a high-risk invasive procedure involving complex factors such as cardiac manipulation and cardiopulmonary bypass, which are often accompanied by physical and psychological complications. The need for cardiac surgery is usually accompanied by fragility and fear on the part of patients, so it is common for symptoms of anxiety and symptoms suggestive of depression to appear or exacerbate in these individuals, which can alter the quality of life of these patients undergoing cardiac surgery. This study aims to assess the presence of symptoms suggestive of depression and anxiety in adult and elderly patients before and after heart surgery. This is a non-controlled prospective cohort study carried out in two hospitals in the municipality of Passo Fundo/RS. Data was collected at three different points in time, pre-surgery, post-surgery during hospitalization and three months after the surgical procedure, using the Clinical Socio-demographic Questionnaire, the Anxiety and Depression Rating Scale and the SF-36 Quality of Life Questionnaire. A descriptive and inferential analysis of the data was carried out. The significance level will be 0.05. The results of this study were that patients undergoing heart surgery in the institutions evaluated had the following predominant socio-demographic characteristics: average age 59.9 years, male 44 (62.9%), white 60 (85.7), married 47 (67.1%), Catholic 57 (81.4), professional farmer 33 (47.1%), retired 48 (68.6%). They came from cities in the interior of Rio Grande do Sul 60 (85.7), from urban areas 42 (60.0%). Among the clinical characteristics, the most frequent comorbidity was Systemic Arterial Hypertension 47 (67.1%), with a length of hospital stay of 12.5 days, three days in the Intensive Care Unit, with surgery to replace the heart valve being the most common procedure 40 (57.1). After analyzing the data, it was concluded that patients had a higher degree of anxiety and depression in the preoperative phase, with a statistically significant reduction in these symptoms three months after the procedure (phase III). With regard to quality of life, it can be concluded that cardiac surgery has a positive impact on patients' quality of life in all the domains assessed, which is statistically significant, especially three months after the procedure.

Keywords: 1. Anxiety. 2. Depression. 3. cardiovascular surgical procedures.

LIST OF SYMBOLS

≥	Greater than or equal to
>	Larger
<	Minor
≤	Less than or equal to
±	Standard Deviation
%	Percentage
/	Division/bar

1 INTRODUCTION

Technological advances in the health sector, among other factors, have made it possible to increase the population's longevity. However, this demographic reality has resulted in an increase in the prevalence of chronic diseases, requiring health professionals to have extensive knowledge and to adapt their care. In this group, we can mention the various cardiovascular diseases, such as coronary syndromes, valvular heart disease, aneurysms, hypertension, among others, which have a high incidence in the population, especially in adults and the elderly. Many of these conditions require surgical treatment, and cardiac surgery can optimize the treatment of these patients, improving their quality of life.

The indication for heart surgery is an important event in anyone's life. It indicates the need to correct a disease which, if left untreated, will lead to physical suffering and even death. Symptoms such as anxiety and depression can therefore be observed in the period from the discovery of the need for major surgery, such as heart surgery, to the moment the surgery is performed and its aftermath.

Knowing the potential emotional, affective and behavioral effects that the indication of cardiac surgery brings to patients, especially in the adult and elderly population, we see the need to identify the symptoms of anxiety and symptoms suggestive of depression that arise in the perioperative period in this population, as well as to evaluate the impact on the quality of life of these patients, thus aiming to find ways to help these individuals cope with this very difficult time in their lives.

We believe that understanding the symptoms suggestive of depression and anxiety in the adult and elderly population undergoing cardiac surgery will help us to understand these changes, as well as alternatives for coping that will benefit this population in their daily routine. These findings could be applied by health services, bringing greater comfort to these patients, helping them to better understand their disease process and thus minimizing their emotional suffering.

This study was carried out at the two main hospitals in the northern region of Rio Grande do Sul, located in the municipality of Passo Fundo. These hospitals are considered to be a reference in healthcare for the entire population of the region, especially in the area of cardiology. One of the hospitals where the data for this study was collected is a highly complex cardiology hospital and a regional reference in cardiac surgery. The other hospital involved in this study is a hospital in constant growth and development, with its cardiac surgery service having just been set up.

This dissertation is made up of two scientific papers related to the same study. The first describes the clinical and sociodemographic aspects related to patients undergoing cardiac surgery and the presence of anxiety and symptoms suggestive of depression. The second article seeks to provide data on the sociodemographic characteristics of patients undergoing cardiac surgery in relation to their quality of life.

2 LITERATURE REVIEW

2.1 *Introduction*

Population ageing is a worldwide phenomenon, with an increase in life expectancy, which makes it possible to improve the population's living conditions. However, the aging process presents numerous health, social and economic problems experienced by elderly individuals. Thus, we can see that the diseases associated with old age are not part of the normal ageing process, but occur because the functional losses resulting from ageing have led to their appearance (BATTAGIN; CANINEU, 2008).

Chronic heart disease affects millions of people worldwide and is one of the main public health problems due to its high morbidity and mortality rate and repercussions on life (OLIVEIRA et al., 2012). The disease can be treated clinically or surgically, both of which aim to restore the heart's functional capacity in order to reduce symptoms and allow the individual to return to normal activities. Surgery is performed when the probability of a useful life is greater with surgical treatment than with clinical treatment (GALDEANO et al., 2006).

Cardiovascular diseases are related to the growing number of patients who have to undergo cardiac surgery. Such interventions directly affect physical, productivity, social and emotional issues, as well as bringing consequences that can lead to difficult changes in behavior and lifestyle habits, compromising the quality of life of these patients (CUSTÓDIO; GASPARINO, 2013). Psychological factors such as depression and anxiety are related to the development, manifestation and progression of coronary artery disease (FURUYA et al., 2013).

Recent advances in medicine and rigorous patient selection have contributed to an increase in the number of indications for coronary artery bypass graft surgery in the elderly (BATTAGIN; CANINEU, 2008). Therefore, the discovery of coronary disease can be interpreted by the patient, most of the time, as synonymous with loss of health and functional incapacity (VILA; ROSSI; COSTA, 2008).

2.2 *Cardiac surgery and its implications*

Surgery is a complex procedure that involves alterations to various physiological mechanisms, such as contact with drugs and materials that can be harmful to the body, and also imposes a great deal of organic stress (DANTAS; AGUILLAR, 2001). Patients with heart disease require attention from the health team as a whole, since, in addition to the incidence and severity of the disease, social and environmental factors need to be known in order to intervene professional. Faced with this scenario, the author considers it important to seek out knowledge and, to this end, those who are co-responsible for the best results in heart surgery, such as nurses, doctors, perfusionists, physiotherapists and others, are becoming increasingly specialized and dedicated (CARVALHO; MEMEDE; ARAÙJO, 2011).

Ferreira and Veigas (2004) state that heart surgery is a high-risk invasive procedure which targets a vital organ, the heart. Thus, patients who undergo this type of surgery need greater care from the entire multi-professional team during the post-operative period, as the way in which they are approached will contribute to achieving satisfactory results or not, resulting in an increase or decrease in the morbidity and mortality rate (FERREIRA; VEIGAS, 2004). The heart is an organ with great cultural significance, it is the most symbolically charged organ, closely related to the center of emotions, life and death. This significance of the heart influences the way we see events, especially life-threatening illnesses such as heart disease (FERREIRA; VEIGAS, 2004; VARGAS; MAIA; DANTAS, 2006).

Adequate preoperative preparation is fundamental for successful surgical treatment and the team must not ignore knowledge of the patient's previous data (CARVALHO; MEMEDE; ARAÙJO, 2011). It is important for the healthcare team to be aware of the difficulties faced by patients and their families during hospitalization and after discharge (DANTAS; AGUILLAR, 2001).

The patient needs intensive post-operative care in order to preserve a good recovery. The same author states that the postoperative period begins in the operating room and has an early phase, which is the period between the end of the operation and full recovery of consciousness, and a late phase, which is known as the immediate postoperative period, i.e. the period when organic functions are still unstable and covers the first twenty-four hours (CARVALHO; MEMEDE; ARAÙJO, 2011).

Planning a follow-up program for cardiac patients becomes essential and more economical, thus reducing morbidity and mortality and promoting an improvement in the quality of life of these patients (AIKAWA et al., 2014). In the hospital setting, there are constant questions from patients and their families about the recovery process of patients who have undergone heart surgery. The author reports that returning home after hospital discharge is a time of anxiety for patients and their families, since, outside hospital, they feel unprotected from the constant vigilance of the healthcare team, perceiving hospital discharge as a threat to their health (CARVALHO; MEMEDE; ARAÙJO, 2011).

For a good quality cardiac surgery service, it is essential that patients, during hospitalization and especially after discharge, have conscious and competent follow-up by the entire healthcare team. Thus, the planned, systematized, competent and responsible care offered to patients during all the operative phases and adequate outpatient follow-up through education contribute to better and faster rehabilitation (CARVALHO; MEMEDE; ARAÙJO, 2011).

Historically, the literature has shown that the results of coronary artery bypass grafting have been measured in terms of mortality and morbidity; however, it is now well established that coronary artery bypass grafting is a multi-professional phenomenon that is not entirely explained by medical factors.

For this reason, in addition to studying mortality and morbidity after coronary artery bypass graft surgery, many recent studies have identified that it is important to investigate various physical, psychological and social variables that have a significant impact on the postoperative adjustment to coronary artery bypass graft surgery (HAWKES et al., 2006).

2.3 Anxiety

Heart disease and its surgical treatment can represent a new reality that disrupts the patient's self-image. The threat to their health also causes anxiety due to their physical state. The literature lacks studies on anxiety and depression in this group of patients, especially in the preoperative period. The vast majority of studies on this subject only evaluate patients in the post-operative period.

The psychological disorder that most concerns health professionals is anxiety, which is characterized by a transitory emotional state involving psychological conflicts and unpleasant feelings of tension, anguish and suffering (CHEIK et al., 2003). The experience of undergoing heart surgery can be stressful and cause anxiety, which is understandable given the complexity of this surgery, which is a critical event in the lives of patients and their families (TORRATI, 2009).

Anxiety is defined as a great physical and psychological discomfort, being a vague and uncomfortable feeling of discomfort or fear, accompanied by an autonomic response; a feeling of apprehension caused by the anticipation of danger. According to the author, it is a warning signal that draws attention to imminent danger and allows the individual to take measures to deal with the threat. The author also reports that, for the diagnosis of anxiety, some factors may be related such as: threat of death, threat of change in health status, threat of change in the environment (VARGAS; MAIA; DANTAS, 2006).

Anxiety can be understood as a human response to the unknown or caused by a lack of knowledge about the procedure (NOVAES; ROMANO; LAGE, 1996). However, increased anxiety in the pre-operative period can lead to depression in these adult and elderly patients, with alterations in their recovery in the post-operative period (GARBOSSA et al., 2009).

Moerman et al.(1996) advocate the use of anxiety assessment questionnaires for all surgical patients during the preoperative assessment, especially patients with heart disease, who need special attention. They also point out that this practice could select patients who are more likely to present anxious or depressive symptoms in the peri-operative period, thus requiring more in-depth care from the multi-professional team.

Of all the diagnoses made in the preoperative period of heart surgery, anxiety is one of the most common (VARGAS; MAIA; DANTAS, 2006). Symptoms such as fatigue, insomnia, shortness of breath, tachycardia, anorexia and decreased libido can result from both physical and mental illness, often confusing the medical diagnosis during the patient's assessment (CHEIK et al., 2003; GARBOSSA et al., 2009; MARCOLINO et al., 2007). However, anticipation of pain, separation from family, loss of independence, fear of becoming disabled, fear of the surgical procedure and of death are factors that often trigger anxiety symptoms during this period (VARGAS; MAIA; DANTAS, 2006).

Anxiety can influence patients' response to surgical treatment and have negative effects on post-operative recovery. The same authors report that high levels of anxiety before the surgical procedure are associated with post-operative depression, early recovery and exacerbation of pain. In addition, moderate levels of preoperative anxiety can help patients prepare for surgery and reduce the stress of the situation (VARGAS; MAIA; DANTAS, 2006).

Anxiety and depression are the psychiatric disorders most associated with physical illnesses and found in the post-operative period (CHEIK et al., 2003; LIMA et al., 2010). It is also important to note that depressive symptoms can appear as a result of various pathologies, while taking various medications, or after the onset of other psychiatric illnesses (CHEIK et al., 2003).

It is considered that reducing patient anxiety and preparing for surgery are important for reducing fears such as: fear of the unknown, fear of death and fear of altering their body image, which contribute to patient anxiety in the preoperative period (VARGAS; DANTAS; GOIS, 2005).

Identifying how patients face and deal with the situation of awaiting heart surgery is an important aspect for the professionals who assist them. Knowing about the presence of defense mechanisms and how the patient responds to the situation are important both pre- and post-operatively. According to the author, there is a range of anxiety that is considered desirable. However, a high level of anxiety can lead the patient to be apathetic and a low level of anxiety can cause a lack of introversion, making it difficult for professionals to understand and guide them through the situation (NOVAES; ROMANO; LAGE, 1996).

2.4 Depression

According to Pinton et al. (2006), surgical trauma and the transient losses that surgery entails can be associated with a stress reaction. In some cases, surgery triggers depression in people who are predisposed to it or who already have some degree of depression, which can increase in the immediate post-operative period and decrease to previous levels after months (PIGNAY-DEMARIA et al., 2003). According to Pinton et al. (2006), depression is a predictive factor of readmission, poorer quality of life and a greater number of cardiac events in the long term. Recognizing and treating depression can reduce morbidity and subsequent mortality.

Some degree of depression affects at least 30% of patients hospitalized with coronary artery disease, and is associated with an increased risk of mortality and depression in the first few years after hospital discharge. Despite its consequences for prognosis and quality of life, depression is underdiagnosed and undertreated in cardiac patients (LESPÉRANCE; FRASURE-SMITH, 2000).

According to Pinton et al. (2006), patients undergoing coronary artery bypass grafting should be assessed for depression and treated if necessary, since it can be associated with postoperative complications. Studies carried out over the last decade have documented an increase in the prevalence of depression among patients with manifestations of coronary artery disease (PINTON et al., 2006). In addition, depression predicts important future cardiac events (ALEXANDER; GLASSMAN; SHAPIRO, 1998).

However, depression is usually not recognized, diagnosed and treated in general health services. This is mainly because depressed patients' complaints are often somatic, such as various pains and undefined malaise (LIMA et al., 2005). Consequently, a significant number of depressed patients fail to receive an adequate therapeutic approach, which can significantly alter the course of heart disease and increase the risk of death (PINTON et al., 2006; TANAJURA et al., 2002). Some variables have been identified as possible factors in the development and progression of heart disease, such as acute and chronic stress, hostility, depression, social support and socioeconomic status. Recognizing and treating psychosocial stress in patients with coronary artery disease can reduce subsequent morbidity and mortality (PINTON et al., 2006).

According to Pignay-Demaria et al. (2003), depression is associated with the risk of cardiovascular disease, regardless of the classic risk factors, both for healthy patients and for those with coronary artery disease. Among patients with coronary artery disease, the risk of cardiac mortality is two to four times higher in those with depression (SHERWOOD et al., 2005).

In addition to the consequences of depression on the patient's state of health, they can become hostile and uncooperative with the team (LIMA et al., 2005; PINTON et al., 2006). Often, these patients show hopelessness about their state of health, intense feelings of guilt, self-depressive ideas and false negative beliefs. Depressed individuals have a negative and pessimistic view of themselves, the world and the future (LIMA et al., 2005).

The association between depression and the prognosis of patients with coronary artery disease undergoing coronary artery bypass grafting has been addressed in a number of studies, the results of which indicate the need to identify and properly manage those at increased risk of depression. Despite clinical and surgical advances, depression is an important independent predictor of death after coronary artery bypass grafting and should be carefully monitored and treated when necessary (PINTON et al., 2006; SHERWOOD et al., 2005).

In the study carried out by Pinton et al. (2006), there was an association between symptoms of depression and postoperative complications.

The study carried out by Carneiro et al. (2009) highlights the importance of assessing the emotional condition of patients with heart disease undergoing invasive and/or surgical procedures, since the prevalence of emotional alterations is high. According to the study by Pinton et al. (2006), the presence of anxiety and depression can influence the development of cardiovascular damage in previously healthy individuals. Since the 1960s, there have been publications reporting an association between the presence of anxiety and depression and increased morbidity and mortality after coronary artery bypass grafting (PIGNAY-DEMARIA et al., 2003; PINTON et al., 2006).

Identifying patients' feelings in the preoperative period of heart surgery is very important, as it can be a strong predictor of complications in the postoperative period, contributing to an increase in morbidity and mortality in these patients.

2.5 Quality of life

The term "quality of life" has been mentioned a lot and is due to demographic changes, especially longevity and economic growth, which require the adoption of new paradigms in public policy and health practice (CARVALHO, 2013). For Minayo, Hartz and Buss (2000) the term involves many meanings, reflecting knowledge, experiences and values. It is an eminently human notion, which has been taken to mean the degree of satisfaction found in family, social and environmental life, as well as one's own existential aesthetics, reflecting comfort and well-being.

While, for Gois (2009), the term "health-related quality of life" has been used to focus on those aspects of quality of life that are influenced by illness and/or treatment, for Carvalho (2013) quality of life is a highly complex expression and is represented differently for each person or social group.

Research into quality of life began in 1970 with well-being scales (WINKELMANN; MANFROI, 2008). According to the author, new instruments emerged with the aim of generally assessing the most important aspects related to individual quality of life, for example: the *Heath Status Profile* (SF-36), the *Sickness Impact Profile* (SIP) and the *Nothingham Heath Profile* (NHP) (WINKELMANN; MANFROI, 2008).

According to Novato, Grossi and Kiamura (2007), the assessment of the health-related quality of life of individuals with chronic conditions has been the aim of research in the health area and is considered an important indicator of therapeutic results in different clinical situations. By assessing the mechanisms that negatively affect health-related quality of life, it is possible to plan psychosocial interventions that lead to greater well-being (NOVATO; GROSSI; KIMURA, 2007).

To date, few national studies have assessed health-related quality of life in populations of cardiac surgery patients. We therefore set out to discover the health-related quality of life of patients undergoing cardiac surgery.

Anxiety and depression alone can alter quality of life in previously healthy elderly patients, and this effect can extend to patients who are about to undergo or have already undergone cardiac surgery.

In studies carried out in Brazil with patients undergoing coronary artery bypass grafting, the components of the quality of life questionnaire (SF-36) that were most compromised preoperatively were physical aspects, functional capacity and emotional aspects, while after surgery there was an improvement in all the components of the instrument, i.e. in the patients' health-related quality of life (GOIS, 2009).

With the growth of the elderly population and increased longevity, surgical interventions have contributed to increasing survival and prolonging the possible co-morbidities triggered by heart disease. In this way, these actions can intervene in the emotional, physical and social state and, above all, in the quality of life of this population. This can be seen in the study carried out by Nogueira et al. (2008) on quality of life, where major changes were observed in both the physical and mental components, with patients achieving significant improvement in all domains.

When compared to other forms of treatment, coronary artery bypass grafting provides patients with a better quality of life (QoL) (TAKIUTI et al., 2007). However, in the study carried out by Nogueira et al. (2008), all the patients studied showed a progressive improvement in quality of life and an early return to work, regardless of the surgical technique used.

Favarato et al.(2006) observed an increase in the quality of life of patients who underwent different types of therapeutic cardiac surgery, however, patients who underwent coronary artery bypass grafting had a more favorable evolution, corroborating the study by Gois, Dantas and Torrati

(2009), who stated that the participants in their study improved their quality of life six months after coronary artery bypass graft surgery.

According to Favarato et al. (2006), a comparison of quality of life in patients undergoing different cardiac treatments revealed that patients undergoing coronary artery bypass grafting had the worst results in the initial assessment, but at six and twelve months after the procedure there was a progressive improvement, surpassing patients undergoing clinical treatment and angioplasty in almost all dimensions of the quality of life questionnaire (SF-36). Therefore, it can be considered that although surgical patients were the most compromised in their quality of life from the point of view of the physical and mental components, surgery provided a significant increase in quality (FAVARATO et al., 2006).

In the assessment of general health and vitality, both men and women over the age of 65 show the best results in the initial post-operative phase. One hypothesis to be raised is that elderly people cope more easily with the changes resulting from loss, particularly in relation to declining health, and perhaps use mechanisms to adapt to these losses more effectively, with more realistic expectations (FAVARATO et al., 2006).

According to Nogueira et al. (2008), when comparing elderly people aged over and under 65 who had undergone coronary artery bypass graft surgery, there were no marked differences in seven of the eight domains assessed (functional capacity, physical aspect, pain, general state of health, vitality, social aspect, emotional aspect), except in the perception of mental health, in which patients aged under 65 achieved a significant perception of improvement.

For Gois, Dantas and Torrati (2009), the participants in their study had a better HRQoL assessment six months after CABG. According to the components of the SF-36, they correlated positively with the age of the patients, showing that with increasing age there is an improvement in HRQoL.

In the study carried out by Favarato et al. (2006), in the evaluation after six months, the results obtained by the women were very close to those of the men, remaining distant only in terms of vitality, which is a mental component, but which is influenced by the physical components. At 12 months, the women again showed a loss compared to the men, with impairment of both the physical and mental components. In the initial assessment, women showed greater impairment than men in functional capacity, followed by emotional aspects, social aspects, mental health and vitality. Thus, the greatest impairment in women was in mental components (FAVARATO et al., 2006).

For Abelha et al. (2010), only 31% of patients who survived after surgery showed a positive subjective perception of HRQoL six months after discharge. More than half of the patients were dependent in at least one instrumental activity of daily living six months after discharge, which could be seen as an indicator of prolonged convalescence in this group of patients. Despite the limitations found in the study, where it was not possible to compare the quality of life of patients before and after surgery, the study showed high degrees of dependence in instrumental and personal ADL after surgery, these results may be influenced by the presence of comorbidities and concomitant diseases (ABELHA et al., 2010). According to Gois, Dantas and Torrati (2009), men had a better HRQoL before and after CABG than women, but the differences were only statistically significant for general health and pain. In this study, there was no association between HRQoL, schooling and marital status of patients six months after surgery, and it can be concluded that CABG improved the participants' HRQoL.

In terms of functional capacity, males showed significantly better results. In addition, males showed a significant improvement in terms of perception of physical appearance when compared to females in the first six months of follow-up (NOGUEIRA et al., 2008).

In the study carried out by Favarato et al. (2006), the quality of life of patients with coronary artery disease (CAD) who underwent clinical, surgical or angioplasty treatment was evaluated, comparing possible differences between genders. Men had a better quality of life at the beginning, benefiting progressively after six and twelve months of treatment, while women showed an improvement after six months followed by a drop at twelve months.

Quality of life is impaired in patients with severe and stable coronary artery disease. This impairment is accentuated in women and patients with other comorbidities, such as diabetes mellitus, overweight, obesity, uncontrolled hypertension and cardiovascular events or previous percutaneous coronary intervention. There was a higher risk of unfavorable outcomes in women and in patients with previous cardiovascular events or procedure failure after twelve months (MORIEL et al., 2010).

For Ciconelli et al. (1999), women also had a higher risk of impaired quality of life, and the higher risk of events in women could be associated, in part, with the fact that they have more depressive symptoms and poorer psychosocial adjustment to a cardiovascular event.

A study aimed at comparing the quality of life of patients assigned to clinical or surgical treatment during ten years of follow-up revealed that the improvement in quality of life, the reduction in anginal symptoms, the increase in physical activity and the reduction in the use of antianginal drugs was superior in patients treated by surgery only in the first years of follow-up. At the end of the study, there was a return of angina symptoms in patients in the surgical group, compromising their quality of life (ROGERS et al., 1990).

In the study carried out by Takiuti et al. (2007), improvement was observed in all the SF-36 domains and in the three therapeutic options (surgery, angioplasty and clinical treatment). In comparison, surgery offered a better quality of life after four years of follow-up.

Coping strategies for coronary heart disease and coronary artery bypass grafting are based on the presence and support of the family, the quality of inter-family relationships, the use of spiritual resources and participation in rehabilitation programs which, in addition to physical conditioning, enable social interaction (KOERICH et al., 2013).

In relation to age group, there was no significant influence of age groups, for both sexes, on the evolution of quality of life (FAVARATO et al., 2006).

In view of this relevant observation of the need to identify feelings of anxiety and depression in patients before and after cardiac surgery, it is of fundamental importance to optimize patients' complaints and provide them with a better quality of life throughout the perioperative period. The aim of this study is to assess the presence of symptoms suggestive of anxiety and depression in adult and elderly patients before and after heart surgery.

3 SCIENTIFIC PRODUCTION I

ANXIETY AND SYMPTOMS SUGGESTING DEPRESSION IN ADULTS AND ELDERLY SUBJECTS OF CARDIAC SURGERY

Summary

Introduction: Patients undergoing cardiac surgery often experience strong feelings of anguish and anxiety in the preoperative period because it is a highly invasive procedure. Anxiety and symptoms suggestive of depression in the preoperative period can lead to various complications in the postoperative period. **Aim: To** identify the presence of symptoms suggestive of depression and anxiety in patients undergoing cardiac surgery. **Methodology:** This was a non-controlled prospective cohort study carried out in two hospitals in Passo Fundo. Data was collected at three different times, preoperatively, postoperatively during hospitalization and three months after the surgical procedure, using the Sociodemographic Clinical Questionnaire and the Anxiety and Depression Rating Scale. The data was analyzed using descriptive and inferential analysis at a significance level of 0.05. **Results:** The frequency of anxiety symptoms was observed to be 38.6% in phase I, 18.6% in phase II and 8.6% in phase III. In patients undergoing cardiac surgery with symptoms suggestive of depression, we observed a frequency of 12.9% in phase I, 10.0% in phase II and 7.1% in phase III. **Conclusion:** After analyzing the data, patients showed a higher degree of anxiety and depression in the preoperative phase (phase I), with a significant reduction in these symptoms three months after the procedure (phase III).

Keywords: 1. Anxiety. 2. Depression. 3. cardiovascular surgical procedures.

3.1 Introduction

Cardiac surgery is considered to be a major operation, so caring for patients who are to undergo cardiac surgery requires skill and knowledge on the part of all health professionals regarding the possible fears and emotional reactions that patients may have to this situation.

The prospect of undergoing heart surgery frightens any human being, as it is a vital organ, with various cultural beliefs and meanings as an organ that controls life and is responsible for emotions, so heart disease and its surgical treatment can represent a new reality, a restructuring of daily life and a threat to the future (VARGAS; MAIA; DANTAS, 2006).

Anxiety and depression are the psychiatric disorders most associated with physical illnesses (MARCOLINO et al., 2007). Among the psychological diagnoses made in the preoperative period of heart surgery, anxiety is one of the most common symptoms. Anxiety can influence the patient's response to surgical treatment and have negative effects on postoperative recovery (QUINTANA;

KALIL, 2012). Thus, the anticipation of pain, separation from family, loss of independence and fear of death or becoming disabled are factors that trigger anxiety symptoms during this period (MARCOLINO et al., 2007).

According to Quintana and Kalil (2012), high rates of anxiety before heart surgery are associated with postoperative depression, poor recovery and exacerbation of pain. Depression is usually not recognized, diagnosed and treated, mainly because depressed patients' complaints are often somatic, such as various pains and undefined malaise (LIMA et al., 2005).

Symptoms of depression appear in 10% to 20% of patients with clinical illnesses. However, only a third of these cases are diagnosed and 10% to 30% receive treatment (TANAJURA et al., 2002). In addition to the consequences of depression on the state of health, depressed patients become hostile to the team and uncooperative, with feelings of guilt, self-deprecating ideas and a pessimistic outlook, hindering treatment and recovery (LIMA et al., 2005).

Therefore, this study aims to identify the presence of symptoms suggestive of depression and anxiety in patients undergoing cardiac surgery.

3.2 Method

An uncontrolled prospective cohort study of adults and the elderly who underwent cardiac surgery and were followed up three months after the surgical procedure.

The study was carried out in two large hospitals (Hospital A and B) which are a reference point for the city of Passo Fundo and the surrounding region.

Hospital A is a large hospital with 230 beds, located in the northern region of the state of Rio Grande do Sul, Brazil. It is a teaching hospital, with medical residency services and multiprofessional health residencies in physiotherapy, nursing, psychology and pharmacy. It is a hospital with highly complex services in neurology, oncology and cardiology, serving as a reference for municipalities in the southern region of Brazil. It also has a specialized intensive care service, with 18 beds in the adult unit, of which five beds (27%) are available for cardiac and clinical patients, and ten beds in the neonatal unit. The Adult Intensive Care Unit consists of a general intensive care unit (ICU) designed to care for critically ill patients from various medical specialties, including cardiology patients.

Hospital B is a special-sized hospital, with 614 beds, located in the city of Passo Fundo, in the northern region of Rio Grande do Sul. It is a reference in the area of health and teaching, with medical residency and multiprofessional health residency programs. It offers highly complex services in various medical areas, such as neurology, cardiology and transplants. It has an intensive care service with an adult, pediatric, neonatal and cardiology unit. The cardiac intensive care unit has twelve beds for post-cardiac surgery patients and critically ill cardiac patients.

Inclusion criteria: adult and elderly individuals of both sexes undergoing cardiac surgery admitted to two hospitals in the municipality of Passo Fundo. Exclusion criteria: patients with disabilities or severe hearing, speech and/or mental impairment that would interfere with the completion of the questionnaires; current history of treatment for depressive disorders; patients using psychoactive substances; and patients undergoing emergency cardiac surgery and/or non-cardiac surgery.

The study population consisted of 93 adult and elderly individuals of both sexes who had undergone cardiac surgery and were admitted to two hospitals in the municipality of Passo Fundo between May 1st and July 31st 2015. Six patients undergoing emergency cardiac surgery and one patient undergoing non-cardiac surgical reintervention were excluded from the sample. A total of 86 patients were assessed in the pre- and post-operative periods. Of these, eight died, two had complications (strokes) and six dropped out. A total of seventy patients were followed up over three months.

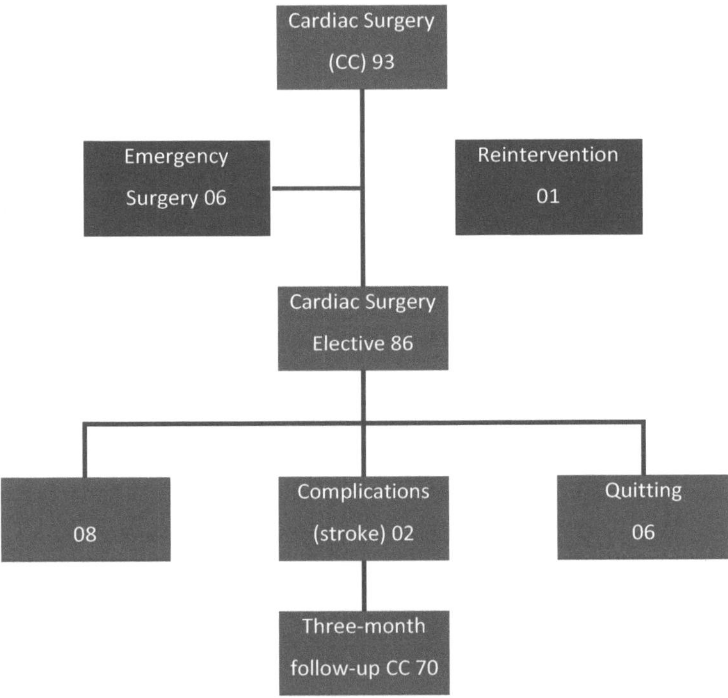

Figure 1- Flowchart, Passo Fundo, 2015

Sampling was carried out by convenience, including all adult and elderly individuals who underwent cardiac surgery at the two hospitals in the city of Passo Fundo between May 1st and July 31st 2015.

This study was approved by the Research Ethics Committee of the University of Passo Fundo. Data collection took place in three stages: pre-surgery (stage I), post-surgery before hospital discharge (stage II) and the late stage - three months after discharge (stage III), which are detailed below.

All participants were informed that the study was divided into three phases, and that the third phase would take place approximately three months after hospital discharge. At the time of phase II, all the participants were scheduled to take part in phase III. On the previously scheduled date, a telephone call was made to confirm and schedule phase III.

All adult and elderly patients with a diagnosis of heart disease and an indication for cardiac surgery who met the inclusion criteria and agreed to take part in the study answered the instruments after individually signing the Informed Consent Form (ICF), which was carried out on hospital premises. Participants were informed of the aim of the study and underwent an initial assessment with the following instruments: Clinical and Sociodemographic Questionnaire; HAD Scale - Assessment of the Level of Anxiety and Depression. All the instruments were essential for checking the inclusion and exclusion criteria. The questionnaires took forty minutes to complete.

All the instruments used in the research are described below:

Clinical and sociodemographic questionnaire: identification of clinical aspects including age, gender, education, profession, marital status, family income, city, residence in rural or urban areas, underlying pathology, medication used, type of surgery performed, cardiopulmonary bypass and cardiopulmonary bypass time, length of hospital stay, duration of illness. This data was collected in the form of a questionnaire answered during the interview with the patients.

Hospital Anxiety and Depression Scale (HAD) - Assessment of the Level of Anxiety and Depression: developed by Zigmond and Snaith (1983), and validated in Portuguese by Botega et al. (1995), it is used to detect cases of mood disorders and can be applied by any health professional, not being an instrument exclusively for psychologists. It has been used both for diagnostic screening and to measure the severity of the disorder, showing good acceptability and ease of answering. Its use can detect cases of mood disorders that may go unnoticed in conventional assessments. The Hospital Anxiety and Depression Scale (HAD) consists of 14 items, divided into two subscales (anxiety and symptoms suggestive of depression), with seven items aimed at assessing anxiety (HAD-A) and seven items for symptoms suggestive of depression (HAD-D). Each item can be scored from zero to three, giving a maximum score of 21 points for each subscale. The cut-off points indicated by Zigmond and Snaith and recommended for both subscales were adopted: HAD-A without anxiety, 0 to 8; with anxiety$\geq$ 9; HAD-D without depression 0 to 8; with depression ≥ 9.

In phase II, adult and elderly patients undergoing cardiac surgery were reassessed prior to discharge from the ICU, around three to five days after surgery, using the following tests: Hospital Anxiety and

Depression Scale (HAD) (described above). The time taken to apply the instruments was approximately twenty minutes.

This stage took place three months after the surgical procedure and was previously scheduled at the time of the phase II evaluation, with telephone calls made a few days beforehand to confirm. It consisted of a reassessment for the continuation of the study, in which adult and elderly patients undergoing cardiac surgery answered the following test: Hospital Anxiety Scale and Depression (HAD) (described above). The test was administered on the premises of the hospitals involved in the study or by telephone, according to the patient's preference. At the Hospital da Cidade de Passo Fundo, the phase III assessment took place in the cardiology outpatient clinic, located in the basement of the hospital, entered via Rua Uruguai. At the Sao Vicente de Paulo Hospital, this assessment took place in the cardiology outpatient clinic, which is accessed via Rua XV de Novembro. The phase III evaluations at both hospitals were carried out after the medical re-evaluation appointment, thus taking advantage of the patient's commute, so there were no extra costs. The time allotted for applying the instruments was twenty minutes.

The team was made up of one professional and two Scientific Initiation scholarship holders from the Psychology course, two resident physiotherapists from the Multiprofessional Cardiology Residency Program and a volunteer physiotherapist. The first was the researcher responsible for the study, who, together with the other interviewers, carried out the data collection, applying the instruments: Clinical and Sociodemographic Questionnaire, Hospital Anxiety and Depression Scale (HAD) before, after and three months after the procedure.

The interviewers were trained and qualified to apply the questions. They received training lasting eight hours, when the research project was presented, along with the objectives, inclusion and exclusion criteria, methodology and research design. The method of approaching the subjects, conducting the interviews and explaining in detail how to apply the questionnaires to collect the data were discussed. The researcher supervised all stages of the research.

The data was coded and entered by the researcher into an MS Excel spreadsheet. Categorical variables were described as absolute and relative frequency. Numerical variables were described as mean ± standard deviation or median ($percentile_{25}$ - $percentile_{75}$), depending on whether they had a normal or non-normal distribution. Variation in anxiety and depression scores over time was assessed using analysis of variance for repeated measures. Tests with a probability value < 0.05 were considered statistically significant.

This study and the informed consent form were submitted to the Research Ethics Committee of the University of Passo Fundo, RS (in accordance with Resolution 466/12 of the National Health Council CNS of December 12, 2012, on the participation of people in research) and were approved by the

Research Committees of the Passo Fundo City Hospital and the Sao Vicente de Paulo Hospital. The subjects who agreed to take part in the research signed the Informed Consent Form (ICF). The study was approved by the Research Ethics Committee of the University of Passo Fundo - RS, under protocol numberol.029.446.

3.3 Results

Of the 93 patients who underwent cardiac surgery between May 1 and July 31, 2015 at the institutions under study, seven patients were excluded from the sample because they met the exclusion criteria, six due to emergency surgery and one due to reintervention. Thus, 86 patients corresponded to elective surgery and were included in the sample. Of these, two (2.3%) were excluded due to in-hospital strokes, eight patients (9.3%) due to death, and six (7.0%) due to loss to follow-up, with 70 (81.4%) completing the three-month follow-up.

Table 1 describes the sociodemographic characteristics of the study population. The average age of the population was 59.9 years (± 14.0). Of these, 62.9% were male. Most of the patients were married. Most of the patients who underwent heart surgery came from different cities in Rio Grande do Sul (85.7%), only 10.0% lived in Passo Fundo and 4.3% came from Santa Catarina. There was a predominance of people living in urban areas (60.0%). On the other hand, the most common occupation was farmer (47.1%). Of the participants, 68.6% are retired. The most common religion was Catholicism, 81.4%. The most prevalent color was white, 88.6%.

Table 1 - Socio-demographic characteristics of the study population (n=70), Passo Fundo, 2015.

Variable	Statistics	
Average age *(years)*		59.9± 14.0
Male		44 (62,9%)
Marital status	Single	5 (7,1%)
	Married	47 (67,1%)
	Divorced	6 (8,6%)
	Viùvo	9 (12,9%)
	Other	3 (4,3%)
Origin	Passo Fundo	7 (10,0%)
	Other - RS	60 (85,7%)
	SC	3 (4,3%)
Zone	Rural	28 (40,0%)

	Urban	42 (60,0%)
Profession	Farmer	33 (47,1%)
	Home	6 (8,6%)
	Other	31 (44,3%)
Retired		48 (68,6%)
Religion	Catholic	57 (81,4%)
	Evangelical	8 (11,4%)
	Other	5 (7,1%)
Color	White	62 (88,6%)
	Black	7 (10,0%)
	Indigenous	1 (1,4%)

RS: Rio Grande do Sul; SC: Santa Catarina. Values expressed mean ± standard deviation and absolute and relative frequency

Table 2 describes the clinical characteristics of the study population. Of the patients who underwent cardiac surgery, the most prevalent underlying diseases were Diabetes, Hypertension, Coronary Artery Disease (CAD) and a smaller number of patients had COPD and Chronic Renal Failure. 58.6% of the patients had valvular heart disease. Of the patients evaluated, 11.4% were smokers and 25.7% were former smokers.

Table 2 - Clinical characteristics of the study population (n=70), Passo Fundo, 2015.

Variable	Statistics
Diabetes	22 (31,4%)
Hypertension	47 (67,1%)
COPD	5 (7,1%)
IRC	7 (10,0%)
DAC	30 (42,9%)
Valvulopathy	41(58,6%)
Smoking	
	No 44 (62.9%)
	Yes 8 (11.4%)

	Former smoker 18 (25.7%)
Pre-depression	18 (25,7%)
Depression in treatment	6 (8,6%)
Time since diagnosis (years)	1,0 (0 - 1,0)

COPD: Chronic Obstructive Pulmonary Disease; CRF: Chronic Renal Insufficiency; CAD: Coronary Artery Disease.

Values express absolute and relative frequency or median (P25 - P75).

Table 3 describes the characteristics of the surgical procedures performed on the study population. Among the most frequently performed procedures, 35.7% underwent coronary artery bypass grafting (CABG). Regarding CPB time, we observed a median of 77.0 minutes (17.5 - 95.5) in the patients evaluated (n=9). This low number of patients evaluated in relation to CPB was due to a difficulty encountered in collecting data from patients undergoing cardiac surgery in one of the hospitals evaluated, as this information (CPB time) is not available in the patient's medical records. In this way, we only assessed the CPB time of patients undergoing cardiac surgery at one of the hospitals evaluated. The median length of hospital stay was 12.5 days (9.0 - 17.0) and the median length of stay in specialized intensive care units (ICU) was 3.0 days (3.0 -5.0).

Table 3 - Characteristics of surgical procedures (n=70), Passo Fundo, 2015.

Variable	Statistics
Type of Procedure***	
Revascularization (CABG)	25 (32,9%)
Valve replacement	40 (52,6%)
Other Cardiac Surgeries	11 (14,5%)
CPB time* (minutes)**	77,0 (17,5 - 95,5)
Length of stay (days)**	12,5 (9,0 - 17,0)
ICU time (days)	3,0 (3,0 - 5,0)

ECC: extra-corporeal circulation; ICU: intensive care unit.

*: n=9.

Values express absolute and relative frequency or **median (p25 - p75).

*** six patients underwent two procedures

Table 4 describes the prevalence of anxiety and depression in the study population. Among the patients assessed in phase I (preoperative), 38.6% had symptoms of anxiety. In phase II (post-surgery), 18.6% still had symptoms of anxiety and in phase III (follow-up three months after the procedure), only 8.6% had symptoms suggestive of anxiety. As seen and described in Figure 1, we can see a statistically significant reduction in anxiety symptoms in individuals undergoing cardiac surgery between phases I and III and between phases II and III. Table 4 also shows that among the patients who underwent cardiac surgery in phase I (preoperative), 12.9% had symptoms suggestive of depression, while in phase II (postoperative), 10.0% had such symptoms and, in the three-month follow-up after the surgical procedure (phase III), only 7.1% had symptoms related to depression. As shown in Figure 2, we can also see a reduction in symptoms suggestive of depression between phases II and III and phases I and III, which were statistically significant ($p<0.05$).

Table 4 - Prevalence of anxiety and depression in the study population (n=70), Passo Fundo, 2015

Variables	Pre-Proc.	Post-Proc.	3m follow-up
	n(%)	n(%)	n(%)
Anxiety (HAD) - Yes	27 (38,6)	13 (18,6)	6(8,6)
Depression (HAD) - Yes	9 (12,9)	7 (10,0)	5(7,1)

HAD: Hospital Anxiety and Depression Scale. Values express absolute and relative frequency

Figure 1 shows a significant variation in anxiety symptoms over time ($p<0.001$). There was a non-statistically significant reduction in the score post-surgery compared to baseline, mean difference 0.81 (95%CI -0.29 - 1.91, p=0.148), there was a statistically significant reduction at three months follow-up compared to post-surgery, mean difference 2.00 (95%CI 1.14 - 2.85, $p<0.001$), also significantly lower than the baseline score, mean difference 2.81 (95%CI 0.29 - 3.86, $p<0.001$).

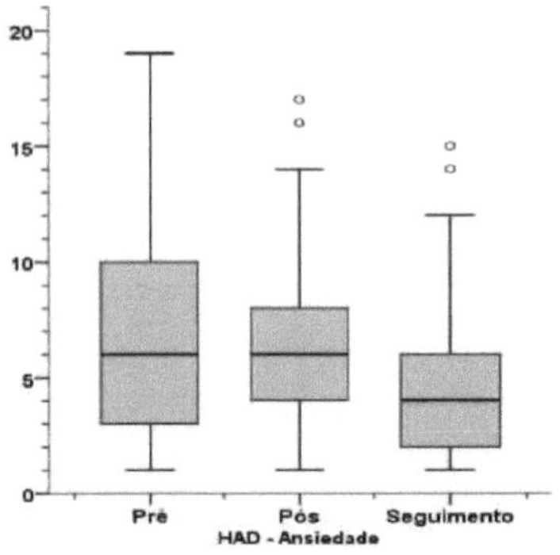

Figura 2 Average score of Anxiety symptoms - HAD Scale, Passo Fundo, 2015

Figure 2 shows a significant variation in symptoms suggestive of depression over time ($p<0.001$). There was a non-statistically significant reduction in the score post-surgery compared to baseline, mean difference - 0.34 (95%CI -1.24 - 0.55, p=0.45), there was a statistically significant reduction at three months follow-up compared to post-surgery, mean difference 1.62 (95%CI 0.68 - 2.57, p =0.001), also significantly lower than the baseline score, mean difference 1.28 (95%CI 0.42 - 2.15, p=0.004).

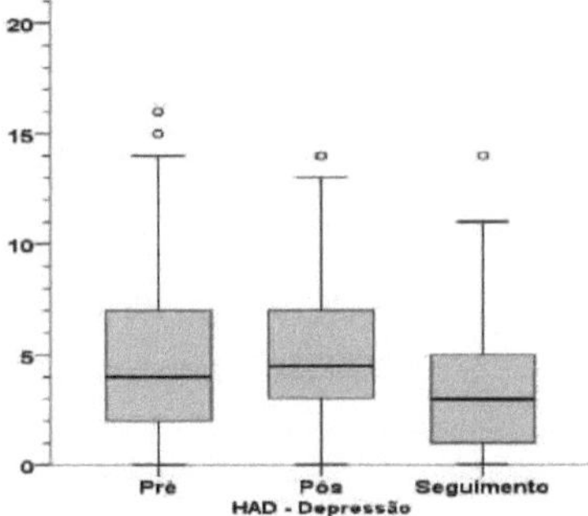

Figura 3 - Average score of symptoms suggestive of depression - HAD Scale, Passo Fundo, 2015

3.4 Discussion

One of the aims of this study was to describe the sociodemographic profile of patients undergoing heart surgery and its relationship with symptoms of anxiety and depression. Different variables were analyzed, such as: gender, age, color, profession, marital status and origin of these patients.

Of the patients assessed during this period, there was a predominance of males. Similar figures were found in the studies carried out by (CARNEIRO et al., 2009; CSERÉP et al., 2014; LIMA et al., 2005; LOURES et al., 2000; TONIAL; MOREIRA, 2011). However, the study carried out by Marcolino et al. (2007) found a predominance of females in their sample (54.4%), as did the study carried out by Tanajura et al. (2002), which found a predominance of females (52.4%) among patients undergoing cardiac surgery. Sherwood et al. (2005) observed a predominance of females in patients with depression 55% and a predominance of males in patients without depression 76%.

The average age found in this study was 59.9±14.0 years, similar to the data found by (CARNEIRO et al., 2009; SHERWOOD et al., 2005; TONIAL; MOREIRA, 2011). Lower values of 41.1±15.34 and 43.9±12.5 years were found, respectively, in the studies carried out by (MARCOLINO et al., 2007; TANAJURA et al., 2002). Meanwhile, the average age of 74.5 years was found in the study by (LOURES et al., 2000), higher than the values found in the other studies.

With regard to marital status, this study found that the majority of patients undergoing cardiac surgery were married, 47 (67.1%), corroborating the study by (CARNEIRO et al., 2009; MARCOLINO et al., 2007) in which 50.6% and 75.0% of patients were married, respectively, and contradicting the study by (TANAJURA et al., 2002), in which the majority of patients undergoing cardiac surgery were unmarried, 52.4%.

The analysis of professional categories identified that most of the individuals were farmers. It was also observed that the majority of patients undergoing heart surgery are retired, contrary to the study carried out by (TANAJURA et al., 2002) in which it was observed that only 23.8% are retired, with a predominance of professionally active people 66.7%, as well as in the study carried out by (LIMA et al., 2005) in which a low prevalence of retired people 6.7% and a higher number of active workers 54.2% were observed.

Evaluating emotional processes in patients undergoing coronary artery bypass grafting with cardiopulmonary bypass, Plotek et al. (2015) found a predominance of professionally active patients (59.6%) and, among the inactive patients, none received pensions due to heart disease. Contrary to the data found in this study, where there was a predominance of retired patients.

From the clinical characteristics of the study population, it was observed that of the patients undergoing cardiac surgery, the majority are hypertensive, diabetic and have CAD, and a small number of patients have COPD and CRF. Similar data was found in studies carried out by (ANDERSON et al., 2011; LOURES et al., 2000; SHERWOOD et al., 2005; TONIAL; MOREIRA, 2011).

It can be seen that the prevalence of smoking among patients undergoing cardiac surgery has decreased compared to other studies described in the literature. We found that only 11.4% of patients are active smokers, while the majority of patients are not smokers. Only the study carried out by Anderson et al. (2011) described a relatively low number of smoking patients - 17.4%. The other data found in the literature describe a higher number of smokers - 48% and 30.7%, respectively, as described by (LOURES et al., 2000; TONIAL; MOREIRA, 2011).

We can see that the majority of surgeries were elective, corroborating the studies carried out by (ALMEIDA et al., 2003; BIANCO et al., 2005; MESQUITA et al., 2008; TONIAL; MOREIRA, 2011).

In the present study, we observed a median hospital stay of 12.5 days, a longer period than the studies published in the literature, which ranged from

8 and 11 days (BIANCO et al., 2005; CSERÉP et al., 2014; MESQUITA et al., 2008; TONIAL; MOREIRA, 2011).

This study showed that patients undergoing cardiac surgery had a high level of anxiety and symptoms suggestive of depression in the preoperative period, with a statistically significant reduction in these symptoms in the postoperative period, especially at the three-month follow-up. In the study carried out by Carneiro et al. (2009), anxiety and depression were assessed using the HAD scale in the preoperative period in patients undergoing invasive cardiac procedures. It was shown that patients with heart disease undergoing invasive and/or surgical cardiac procedures such as electrophysiological studies, pacemaker implantation and coronary artery bypass grafting had a high prevalence of anxiety and depression, and that this level of anxiety was higher in patients undergoing electrophysiological studies. In the study carried out by Pignay-Demaria et al. (2003), it was shown that patients undergoing coronary artery bypass grafting had high levels of anxiety in the preoperative period, corroborating the present study.

According to Dayan and Ricca (2014), coronary artery bypass graft surgery is associated with significant anxiety and depression during convalescence, and patients with higher anxiety and depression scores have a higher risk of being re-hospitalized in the six months following the surgical procedure.

Hawkes et al. (2006) evaluated the outcomes of coronary artery bypass graft surgery and found that patients' anxiety levels increased before surgery, but fell rapidly in the post-operative period. They also indicate that a number of patients undergoing coronary artery bypass grafting are depressed immediately after surgery, returning to preoperative levels at hospital discharge.

Timberlake et al. (1997) evaluated the incidence of depression following coronary artery bypass graft surgery. They found that 50% of patients were significantly depressed eight days after surgery, with a substantial decline to 24% of patients eight weeks after surgery and 22% 12 months after surgery. In the present study, we found symptoms suggestive of depression, at lower levels than those found in the study described above.

The high rate of anxiety in the preoperative period observed in this study is in line with other data found in the literature, such as those described by Carneiro et al.(2009), where a high level of anxiety was observed in the different procedures evaluated, including in 34.4% of patients undergoing a coronary artery bypass graft. In another study by Marcolino et al. (2007), 44.3% of the patients assessed had anxiety and 26.6% had depression. This high frequency of anxiety showed that a considerable proportion of patients have these symptoms, and therefore deserve to receive a more detailed assessment of their mental state before the surgical intervention is carried out.

Another study also assessed the rates of anxiety and depression, using the HAD scale, before and after the angioplasty procedure, evaluating 35 patients. This study found an average of 12.7 patients with anxiety preoperatively and an average of 6.1 patients with anxiety postoperatively. With regard to depression, the average found in the preoperative period was 11.4 patients, while in the postoperative period there were 7.2 patients with depression, both statistically significant (CHAUDHURY; SRIVASTAVA, 2013). These data are in line with the results found in this study.

3.5 Conclusion

The results of this study reinforce the importance of assessing anxiety and symptoms suggestive of depression in patients with heart disease undergoing surgery, since their prevalence is high and can interfere with their treatment and recovery. This study also shows the importance of psychological assessment during hospitalization, as well as the need for psychological intervention and support for patients undergoing cardiac surgery in the pre- and post-operative periods.

3.6 References

ABELHA, F. J. et al. Evaluation of Quality of Life and Mortality in Patients with Severe Cardiac Events in the Postoperative Period. **Rev Bras Anestesiol**, v. 60, n. 3, p. 268-284, 2010.

AIKAWA, P. et al. Cardiac rehabilitation in patients undergoing coronary artery bypass graft surgery. **Rev Bras Med Esporte**, v. 20, n. 1, p. 55-58, 2014.

ALEXANDER, H. .; GLASSMAN, M. D. .; SHAPIRO, P. A. Depression and the Course of Coronary Artery Disease. **Am J Psychiatry**, v. 155, n. 1, p. 4-11, 1998.

ALMEIDA, F. F. et al. Predictors of Hospital Mortality and Severe Per-Operative Complications in Myocardial Revascularization Surgery. **Arq Bras Cardiol**, v. 80, n. nº 1, p. 41-50, 2003.

ANDERSON, A. J. P. G. et al. Predictors of mortality in patients over 70 years of age undergoing coronary artery bypass grafting or valve replacement with cardiopulmonary bypass. **Rev Bras Cir Cardiovasc**, v. 26, n. 1, p. 69-75, 2011.

BAHRAMNEZHAD, F. et al. Quality of Life in Patients Undergoing Percutaneous Transluminal Coronary Angioplasty (PTCA). **Global journal of health science**, v. 7, n. 5, p. 246-50, jan. 2015.

BATTAGIN, A. M.; CANINEU, P. R. Evaluation of functional capacity and depressive symptoms after cardiac surgery. **O Mundo da Saùde Sao Paulo**, v. 32, n. 2, p. 189-197, 2008.

BIANCO, A. C. M. et al. Prospective Risk Analysis in Patients Undergoing Myocardial Revascularization Surgery. **Arquivos Brasileiros de Cardiologia**, v. 85, n. 4, p. 254-261, 2005.

CARNEIRO, A. F. et al. Evaluation of Anxiety and Depression in the Preoperative Period in Patients Undergoing Invasive Cardiac Procedures *. **Rev Bras Anestesiol**, v. 59, n. 4, p. 431-438, 2009.

CARVALHO, A. L. DE O. **Quality of life after coronary artery bypass grafting, angioplasty or clinical treatment: 10-year follow-up**. [s.l.] University of Sao Paulo, 2013.

CARVALHO, L. D. P.; MEMEDE, M. V.; ARAÙJO, M. DOS R. O. Conhecimento de pacientes sobre o processo de auto-cuidado em pós-operatório de cirurgia cardiaca. **Cad. Pesq.**, v. 18, p. 18-25, 2011.

CHAUDHURY, S.; SRIVASTAVA, K. Relation of Depression , Anxiety , and Quality of Life with Outcome after Percutaneous Transluminal Coronary Angioplasty. **The Scientific World Journal**, v. 2013, 2013.

CHEIK, N. C. et al. Effects of physical exercise and physical activity on depression and anxiety in elderly individuals. **R. Bras. Ci. e Mov.**, v. 11, n. 3, p. 45-52, 2003.

CHOINIÈRE, M. et al. Prevalence of and risk factors for persistent postoperative nonangial pain after cardiac surgery : a 2-year prospective multicenter study. **CMAJ**, v. 186, n. 7, p. 213-23, 2014.

CICONELLI, R. M. et al. Translation into Portuguese and validation of the SF-36 (Brazil SF-36) generic quality of life assessment questionnaire. **Rev Bras Reumatol**, v. 39, n. 3, p. 143-50, 1999.

CSERÉP, Z. et al. Self-rated health is associated with the length of stay at the intensive care unit and hospital following cardiac surgery. v. 14, n. 171, p. 1-9, 2014.

CUSTÓDIO, F. M.; GASPARINO, R. C. Quality of Life of Patients in the Postoperative Cardiac Surgery Phase. **Reme: Revista Mineira de Enfermagem**, v. 17, n. 1, p. 130-134, 2013.

DANTAS, R. A. S.; AGUILLAR, O. M. Problems in the recovery of patients submitted to myocardial revascularization surgery: follow-up by nurses during the first month after hospital discharge. **Rev Latino-am Enfermagem**, v. 9, n. 6, p. 31-36, 2001.

DAYAN, V.; RICCA, R. Cardiac rehabilitation after coronary artery bypass grafting. v. 84, n. 4, p. 286-292, 2014.

FAVARATO, M. E. C. DE S. et al. Quality of life in patients with coronary artery disease: comparison between genders. **Rev Assoc Med Bras**, v. 52, n. 4, p. 23641, 2006.

FERREIRA, L. B.; VEIGAS, M. O. **Epidemiological profile of patients undergoing cardiac surgery at the Santa Genoveva Hospital in Goiânia**. [s.l.] Universidade Católiga de Goiàs, 2004.

FURUYA, R. K. et al. Anxiety and depression among men and women who underwent percutaneous coronary intervention. **Rev da Esc de Enferm USP**, v. 47, n. 6, p. 1333-7, dec. 2013.

GALDEANO, L. E. et al. Nursing diagnoses in the perioperative period of cardiac surgery. **Rev Esc Enferm USP**, v. 40, n. 1, p. 26-33, 2006.

GARBOSSA, A. et al. Effects of physiotherapeutic guidance on anxiety in patients undergoing coronary artery bypass graft surgery. **Rev Bras Cardiovasc**, v. 24, n. 3, p. 359-366, 2009.

GOIS, C. F. L. **Health-related quality of life, depression and sense of coherence of patients before and six months after coronary artery bypass grafting**. [s.l.] University of Sao Paulo, 2009.

GOIS, C. F. L.; DANTAS, R. A. S.; TORRATI, F. G. Health-related quality of life before and six months after coronary artery bypass grafting. **Rev Gaûcha Enferm**, v. 30, n. 4, p. 700-707, 2009.

HAWKES, A. L. et al. Outcomes of coronary artery bypass graft surgery. **Vascular Health and Risk Management**, v. 2, n. 4, p. 477-484, 2006.

KOERICH, C. et al. Myocardial revascularization: strategies for coping with the disease and the surgical process. **Acta Paul Enferm**, v. 26, n. 1, p. 8-13, 2013.

LESPÉRANCE; FRASURE-SMITH. Depression in patients with cardiac disease : a practical review. **Journal of Psychosomatic Research**, v. 48, p. 379-391, 2000.

LIMA, F. E. T. et al. Protocol for nursing consultations with patients after coronary artery bypass grafting: influence on anxiety and depression. **Rev Latino-am Enfermagem**, v. 18, n. 3, p. 35-41, 2010.

LIMA, M. S. et al. Depression in clinical and surgical patients admitted to a general hospital. **Arq Ciênc Saùde**, v. 12, n. 2, p. 63-66, 2005.

LOURES, D. R. DA R. L. et al. Cardiac surgery in the elderly. **Rev Bras Cir Cardiovasc**, v. 15, n. 1, p. 1-5, 2000.

MARCOLINO, J. A. M. et al. Measurement of anxiety and depression in preoperative patients. Comparative study. **Rev Bras Anestesiol**, v. 57, n. 2, p. 157166, 2007.

MESQUITA, E. T. et al. Quality of Care Indicators in Revascularization Surgery. **Arq Bras Cardiol**, v. 90, n. 5, p. 350-354, 2008.

MINAYO, M. C. DE S.; HARTZ, Z. M. DE A.; BUSS, P. M. Qualidade de vida e saù: um debate necessàrio. **Ciências & Saùde Coletiva**, v. 5, n. 1, p. 7-18, 2000.

MOERMAN, N. et al. The Amsterdam Preoperative Anxiety and Information Scale (APAIS). **Anesth Analg**, v. 82, p. 445-51, 1996.

MONTEIRO, R. et al. Quality of life in focus. **Rev Bras Cardiovasc**, v. 25, n. 4, p. 568-574, 2010.

MORIEL, G. et al. Quality of Life in Patients with Severe and Stable Coronary Atherosclerotic Disease. **Arq Bras Cardiol**, v. 95, n. 6, p. 691-697, 2010.

NOGUEIRA, C. R. S. R. . et al. Quality of Life after Coronary Artery Bypass Grafting with and without Cardiopulmonary Bypass. **Arq Bras Cardiol**, v. 91, n. 4, p. 238-244, 2008.

NOVAES, M. A. F. P.; ROMANO, B. W.; LAGE, S. G. Hospitalization in the ICU. Variables that Interfere in the Emotional Response. **Arq Bras Cardiol**, v. 67, n. 2, p. 99102, 1996.

NOVATO, T. DE S.; GROSSI, S. A. A.; KIMURA, M. Quality of life instrument for young people with diabetes. **Rev Gaûcha Enferm**, v. 28, n. 4, p. 512-519, 2007.

OLIVEIRA, S. K. P. et al. Nursing diagnosis present in adult patients in the postoperative of cardiac surgery. **Rev Enferm UFPI**, v. 1, n. 2, p. 95-100, 2012.

PIGNAY-DEMARIA, V. et al. Depression and Anxiety and Outcomes of Coronary Artery Bypass Surgery. **Ann Thorac Surg**, v. 75, p. 314-21, 2003.

PINTON, F. A. et al. Depression as a risk factor for immediate and late morbidity after coronary artery bypass grafting. **Braz J Cardiovasc Surg**, v. 21, n. 1, p. 68-74, 2006.

PLOTEK, W. et al. Emotional processes in patients undergoing coronary artery bypass graft surgeries with extracorporeal circulation in view of selected indicators of the inflammatory condition. **Med Sci Monit**, v. 21, p. 105-17, jan. 2015.

QUINTANA, J. F.; KALIL, R. A. K. Cardiac surgery: psychological manifestations of the patient in the pre- and postoperative period. **Psicologia Hospitalar**, v. 10, n. 2, p. 16-32, 2012.

ROGERS, W. J. et al. Ten-year follow-up of quality of life in patients randomized to receive medical therapy or coronary artery bypass graft surgery. The Coronary Artery Surgery Study (CASS). **Circulation**, v. 82, n. 5, p. 1647-1658, 1 nov. 1990.

SHERWOOD, A. et al. Impaired endothelial function in coronary heart disease patients with depressive symptomatology. **Journal of the American College of Cardiology**, v. 46, n. 4, p. 656-9, Aug. 16, 2005.

TAKIUTI, M. E. et al. Quality of life after coronary artery bypass grafting, angioplasty or clinical treatment. **Arq Bras Cardiol**, v. 88, n. 5, p. 537-544, 2007.

TANAJURA, D. et al. Prevalence of depression in different groups of inpatients at the University Hospital of Bahia , Brazil. **Rev Bras Psiquiatr**, v. 24, n. 4, p. 182185, 2002.

TIMBERLAKE, N. et al. Incidence and patterns of depression following coronary artery bypass graft surgery. **Journal of Psychosomatic Research**, v. 43, n. 2, p. 197-207, 1997.

TONIAL, R.; MOREIRA, D. M. Clinical-epidemiological profile of patients undergoing coronary artery bypass grafting at the Santa Catarina Institute of Cardiology, Sao José - SC. **Arquivos Catarineses de Medicina**, v. 40, n. 4, p. 42-46, 2011.

TORRATI, F. G. **Anxiety, depression, sense of coherence and stressors in the pre- and postoperative periods of cardiac surgery**. [s.l.] University of Sao Paulo, 2009.

VARGAS, T. V. P.; DANTAS, R. A. S.; GOIS, C. F. L. The self-esteem of individuals who have undergone coronary artery bypass graft surgery. **Rev Esc Enferm USP**, v. 39, n. 1, p. 20-27, 2005.

VARGAS, T. V. P.; MAIA, E. M.; DANTAS, R. A. S. Sentiments of patients in the preoperative period of cardiac surgery. **Rev Latino-am Enfermagem**, v. 14, n. 3, p. 1-6, 2006.

VILA, V. DA S. C.; ROSSI, L. A.; COSTA, M. C. S. Experience of heart disease among adults undergoing coronary artery bypass grafting. **Rev Saùde Pùblica**, v. 42, n. 4, 2008.

WINKELMANN, E. R.; MANFROI, W. C. Quality of life in cardiology. **Rev HCPA**, v. 28, n. 1, p. 49-53, 2008.

4 SCIENTIFIC PRODUCTION II

QUALITY OF LIFE OF ADULT AND ELDERLY PATIENTS UNDERGOING CARDIAC SURGERY

Summary

Introduction: Cardiac surgery is an effective means of treating coronary artery disease. It also improves patients' quality of life. The SF-36 quality of life questionnaire makes it possible to monitor health conditions before and after surgical treatment, and is sensitive to clinical improvement. **Objective: To** assess the impact of heart surgery on the quality of life of adult and elderly patients. **Method:** This is a non-controlled prospective cohort study carried out in two large hospitals in Passo Fundo/RS. Data was collected at three different times, preoperatively, postoperatively during hospitalization and three months after the surgical procedure, using a sociodemographic clinical questionnaire and the SF-36 Quality of Life Questionnaire. A descriptive and inferential analysis of the data was carried out. The significance level was 0.05. **Results:** Functional capacity was 40.0 points pre-surgery, 15.0 points post-surgery and 70.0 points three months post-surgery. In the physical limitation domain, the median score before surgery was zero, the same as in the post-surgery phase, and in the three-month follow-up it was 25.0 points. With regard to pain, the preoperative median was 52.0 points, the postoperative median was 32.0 points and the follow-up median was 62.0 points. As for general state of health, the median before surgery was 80.0 points, after surgery 77.0 points and at follow-up 87.0 points. In terms of vitality, the preoperative median was 50.0 points, which was maintained in the postoperative period and increased to 70.0 points after three months. In the social aspect, the pre-surgery median was 62.5 points, in the post-surgery 50.0 points and in the three-month follow-up 87.5 points. Limitation due to emotional aspects had a median of 33.3 points preoperatively, zero points postoperatively and 100.0 points three months after the procedure. The median score for mental health was 64.0 points preoperatively, 68.0 points postoperatively and 76.0 points at follow-up. **Conclusion:** With regard to quality of life, it can be concluded that cardiac surgery has a positive impact on patients' quality of life in all the domains evaluated, which is statistically significant, especially three months after the procedure.

Keywords: 1. Quality of life. 2. Cardiovascular Surgical Procedures.

4.1 Introduction

Studies have shown a higher incidence of cardiovascular events in the population with depressive symptoms and low quality of life scores, so lifestyle and emotional stress are risk factors for cardiovascular diseases and have been highlighted in the literature (MORIEL et al., 2010).

Cardiovascular diseases are directly related to the growing number of patients who have to undergo cardiac surgery. For the author, such interventions directly affect physical, productivity, social and emotional issues, as well as bringing sequelae, which can lead to difficult changes in behavior and lifestyle habits, compromising the quality of life of patients (CUSTÓDIO; GASPARINO, 2013).

The high prevalence of heart disease in the population has major implications for the postoperative period and the risk of serious cardiac events can be significant for patients undergoing major surgery (ABELHA et al., 2010).

If, on the one hand, the growing technological development of medicine has made it possible to treat various diseases, ensuring greater longevity for the population, on the other hand, it has triggered a process of frailty, in which we see an increase in longevity, often with a poor quality of life. Thus, concern with the concept of quality of life has come to rescue psychological, physical and social aspects, as well as economic ones (MONTEIRO et al., 2010).

Quality of life is undoubtedly one of the most talked about and discussed topics today (MONTEIRO et al., 2010). The global definition of quality of life takes into account the external conditions of life and the subjective experiences of the individual. For the author, it is not an easy task to quantify quality of life. To this end, there are several proposed instruments that have been validated by various studies and translated into Brazilian. These include the *Medical Outcomes Study 36-item Short-form Health*

Survey (SF-36) as a more comprehensive instrument that is well applied to patients with chronic diseases (MORIEL et al., 2010).

Therefore, this study aims to assess the impact of heart surgery on the quality of life of adult and elderly patients.

4.2 Method

This was a non-controlled prospective cohort study of adults and elderly people undergoing cardiac surgery, followed up three months after the surgical procedure, carried out on the premises of two large hospitals in the city of Passo Fundo, in the inpatient unit, in the first phase of collection, corresponding to the preoperative assessment, in the Cardiology Intensive Care Center (CTI) and/or Intensive Care Unit (UTI), corresponding to the second phase of the post-operative assessment, and in the Cardiology outpatient clinic or by telephone, according to the participants' preference, the third phase of the collection, corresponding to three months after the cardiac surgery.

Among the cardiac surgeries performed during this period, 86 patients were included in the sample, consecutively, between May 1st and July 31st, 2015. The sample included all adult and elderly individuals of both sexes who underwent cardiac surgery and were admitted to the two hospitals in the municipality of Passo Fundo/RS. Exclusion criteria were patients with disabilities or severe hearing, speech and/or mental impairment that interfered with the questionnaires; patients who had undergone non-cardiac surgical reintervention; and patients undergoing emergency cardiac surgery.

The study was carried out in accordance with Resolution 466/12 of the National Health Council (CNS) of December 12, 2012. The project was submitted to and approved by the Research Ethics Committee of the University of Passo Fundo, RS (UPF), under protocol number 1.029.446, and approved by the Research Committees of the two hospitals. Participants who agreed to take part in the study signed the Informed Consent Form (ICF).

Data collection was carried out by the researcher and five interviewers (two Psychology undergraduate students, two physiotherapist residents from the Multiprofessional Residency Program (PRM) in cardiology and a volunteer physiotherapist) through individual interviews and consultation of the participants' medical records. Before the procedures began, all the interviewers were trained and qualified to administer the questionnaires. Training sessions were held to clarify doubts and the correct way to use and fill in the sociodemographic questionnaire and the SF-36 scale.

A sociodemographic and clinical characterization tool was used. The data for sociodemographic characterization were date of birth, age, gender, marital status, schooling (in years), profession, professional situation (retired or not), ethnicity, religion, children and salary. Clinical data was collected from medical records: type of surgery, date of hospitalization, date of ICU interaction, CPB time, presence of previous comorbidities.

To assess quality of life, we used the Portuguese version of the generic instrument Medical OutcomesStudy 36 - item Short Form (SF-36), devised by Ware and Sherboune and validated for Portuguese by Ciconelli (1999). This questionnaire is a tool that can be applied to people from the age of 12 and is intended to survey physical and mental health status in individualized clinical practice and in the general population. It is a multidimensional questionnaire made up of 36 items covering eight domains in two main components: the physical component, which involves functional capacity (with ten items), pain (two items), general state of health (five items) and physical aspects (four items). The mental component includes mental health (five items), emotional aspects (three items), vitality (four items), and social aspects (two items), which is assessed by 35 questions. In addition, *there is* one more question to compare the current general state of health with that of one year ago (Table 5). The purpose of the questions was to transform subjective measures into objective data that would allow analysis in a specific, global and reproducible way. The instrument covers the last four weeks.

Table 5 - SF-36 Domains and their respective scope

Domain	Scope

Component Physical	Functional Capacity Physical Aspects Pain General state of health	Presence of a physical limitation Limitation of daily activities Intensity and limitations Self-perception of health
Component Mental	Vitality Social aspect Emotional aspect Mental health	Weakness and tiredness Relationships Emotional interference Depression and anxiety

To evaluate the results, we used the score for each question, which evaluates both the negative aspects (disease/illness) and the positive points (well-being). A low numerical score reflects poor health perception, loss of function and the presence of pain, while a high numerical score reflects good health perception, preserved function and the absence of pain. To evaluate the results, the answers to the items are calculated into their respective components, and these values are normalized on a scale from zero to 100. Lower values reflect a perception of poor health and pain (worse evaluation), while higher values reflect a perception of good health, absence of functional deficits and pain (better evaluation of quality of life).

In data analysis, categorical variables were described as absolute and relative frequency. Numerical variables were described as mean ± standard deviation or median ($percentile_{25}$ - $percentile_{75}$), depending on whether they had a normal or non-normal distribution. To evaluate the variation in quality of life over time, analysis of variance was used in which the time effect (baseline, post-surgery and three-month follow-up) of each of the SF-36 domains was specified as an intra-subject effect. For multiple, pairwise comparisons, simple contrast analysis was used. Tests with a probability value < 0.05 were considered statistically significant.

4.3 Results

Of the 93 patients who underwent cardiac surgery between May 1 and July 31, 2015 at the institutions under study, seven patients were excluded from the sample because they met the exclusion criteria, six due to emergency surgery and one due to reintervention. Thus, 86 patients corresponded to elective surgery and were included in the sample. Of these, eight patients (9.3%) died, two (2.3%) suffered an in-hospital stroke and six (7.0%) were lost to follow-up. 70 (81.4%) completed the three-month follow-up.

Table 6 describes the sociodemographic characteristics of the study population. The average age of the study population was 59.9 years (± 14.0). Of these, 62.9% were male. Of the patients evaluated, 67.1% were married. Of the participants, 48 (68.6%) were retired. The most common religion was Catholic, 57 (81.4%). The most prevalent race was white 62 (88.6%).

Table 6 - Socio-demographic characteristics of the study population (n=70), Passo Fundo, 2015

Variable	Statistics	
Average age *(years)*		59.9± 14.0
Male		44 (62,9%)
Marital status		
	Single	5 (7,1%)
	Married	47 (67,1%)
	Divorced	6 (8,6%)
	Viùvo	9 (12,9%)
	Other	3 (4,3%)
Origin		
	Passo Fundo	7 (10,0%)
	Other - RS	60 (85,7%)
	SC	3 (4,3%)
Retired	Yes	48 (68,6%)
	No	22(31,4%)

RS: Rio Grande do Sul; SC: Santa Catarina.

Values express mean ± standard deviation and absolute and relative frequency.

Table 7 describes the clinical characteristics of the study population. Of the patients who underwent cardiac surgery, the most prevalent underlying diseases were diabetes, hypertension and coronary artery disease (CAD), while fewer had COPD and chronic renal failure. Of the patients evaluated, 11.4% are smokers and 25.7% are former smokers.

Table 7 - Clinical characteristics of the study population (n=70), Passo Fundo, 2015

Variable	n·(%)
Diabetes	
Yes	22 (31,4)

No	48 (68,6)
Hypertension	
Yes	47 (67,1)
No	32 (32,9)
COPD	
Yes	5 (7,1)
No	65 (92,9%)
IRC	
Yes	7 (10,0)
No	63 (90,0)
DAC	
Yes	30 (42,9)
No	40 (57,1)
Smoking	
No	44 (62,9%)
Yes	8 (11,4%)
Former smoker	18 (25,7%)

COPD: Chronic Obstructive Pulmonary Disease; CRF: Chronic Renal Insufficiency; CAD: Coronary Artery Disease.

Values express absolute and relative frequency

Table 8 describes the SF-36 domains pre-surgery, post-surgery and at the three-month follow-up. It was observed that in the post-operative functional capacity, there was a drop in the score compared to the pre-operative, while at the three-month follow-up, there was an increase in the functional capacity score. In the limitation by physical aspects domain, the initial score was zero, maintaining the same value found in the post-operative phase, while in the three months follow-up, the score increased. With regard to pain, there was a worsening of pain in the post-operative period compared to the pre-operative period, with an increase in the pain score at the three-month follow-up. The general state of health worsened in the postoperative period compared to the preoperative period, with an improvement in the score at three months. In terms of vitality, the values found preoperatively were maintained postoperatively, with an improvement at the three-month follow-up. As for the social aspect, there was a worsening of the results in the post-operative period, with an improvement in these values at the three-month follow-up.

With regard to limitation due to emotional aspects, there was a worsening of results in the post-operative period compared to the pre-operative period, with an increase in these values at the three-month follow-up. In terms of mental health, there was an improvement in results at the three-month follow-up compared to the pre- and post-operative periods.

Table 8 - Quality of life pre-surgery, post-surgery and at 3-month follow-up (n=70), Passo Fundo, 2015

	Time		
	Pre-surgery	**Post-surgery**	**Follow-up3 months**
Functional capacity	40,0 (25,0 - 70,0)	15,0 (0 - 35,0)	70,0 (50,0 - 80,0)
Limitation by physical aspects	0 (0 -25,0)	0 (0 - 25,0)	25,0 (0 - 100,0)
Pain	52,0 (30,0 - 62,0)	32,0 (22,0 - 54,2)	62,0 (51,0 - 88,0)
General state of health	80,0 (62,0 - 87,0)	77,0 (57,0 - 87,0)	87,0 (67,0 - 92,0)
Vitality	50,0 (30,0 - 66.2)	50,0 (35,0 - 66,2)	70,0 (50,0 - 80,0)
Social aspects	62,5 (34,3 - 87,5)	50,0 (34,3 - 75,0)	87,5 (62,5 - 100,0)
Limitation by emotional aspects	33,3 (0 - 100,0)	0 (0-66,6 - 66,7)	100,0 (67,0 - 100,0)
Mental Health	64,0 (45,0 - 84,0)	68,0 (44,0 - 80,0)	76,0 (67,0 - 92,0)

Values express median (p_{25} - p_{75})

A value close to zero indicates a poorer quality of life

A value close to 100 indicates a better quality of life

Figure 4 shows a significant variation in the functional capacity domain over time (p<0.001). Despite a significant reduction in the post-surgery score compared to baseline, mean difference 25.4 (95% CI 18.9 - 32.0, p<0.001), there was a recovery at the three-month follow-up, mean difference compared to post-surgery 40.7 (95% CI 32.7 - 48.7, p<0.001), reaching values higher than baseline, mean difference 15.3 (95% CI 7.7 - 22.9, p<0.001).

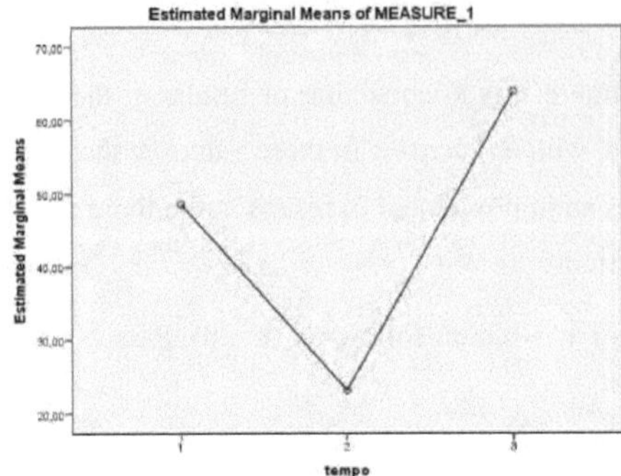

Figura 4 - Functional Capacity - SF-36, Passo Fundo, 2015

Figure 5 shows a significant variation in the physical limitation domain over time (p<0.001). There was a non-statistically significant reduction in the score post-surgery compared to baseline, mean difference 7.1 (95%CI -0.9 - 15.1, p=0.079), a statistically significant increase in the three-month follow-up compared to post-surgery, mean difference 23.6 (95%CI 12.8 - 34.4, p<0.001), also significantly higher than the baseline score, mean difference 16.4 (95%CI 3.1 - 29.8, p=0.017).

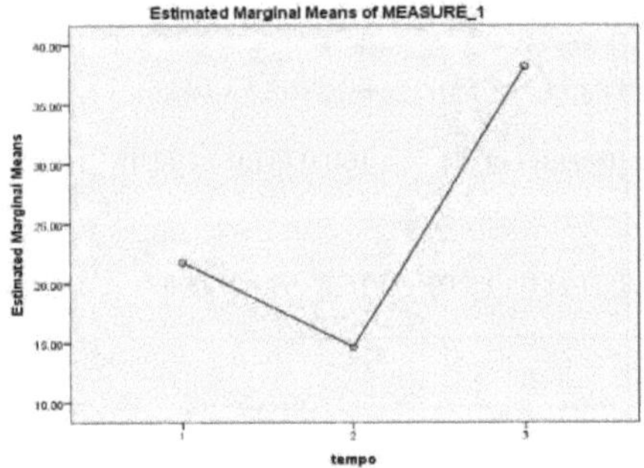

Figura 5 - Limitation by physical aspects - SF-36, Passo Fundo, 2015

Figure 6 shows a significant variation in the pain domain over time (p<0.001). Despite a significant reduction in the post-surgery score compared to baseline, mean difference 13.7 (95% CI 6.0 - 21.3, p=0.001), there was a recovery at the 3-month follow-up, mean difference compared to post-surgery 28.5 (95% CI 22.4 - 34.5, p<0.001), reaching higher values than baseline, mean difference 14.8 (95% CI 6.2 - 23.4, p=0.001).

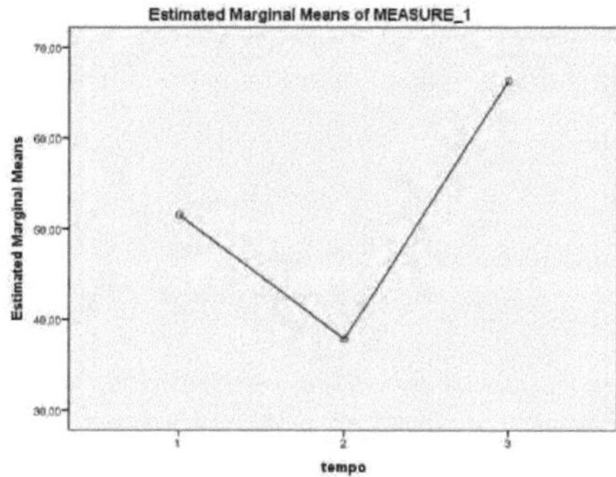

Figura 6 - Pain - SF-36, Passo Fundo, 2015

There was a significant variation in the general health domain over time (p=0.004). There was a non-statistically significant increase in the post-surgery score compared to baseline, mean difference 1.0 (95%CI -5.0 - 6.0, p=0.841), a statistically significant increase in the three-month follow-up compared to post-surgery, mean difference 7.4 (95%CI 2.2 - 12.6, p =0.006), also significantly higher than the baseline score, mean difference 8.0 (95%CI 2.9 - 13.0, p=0.002) (Figure 7).

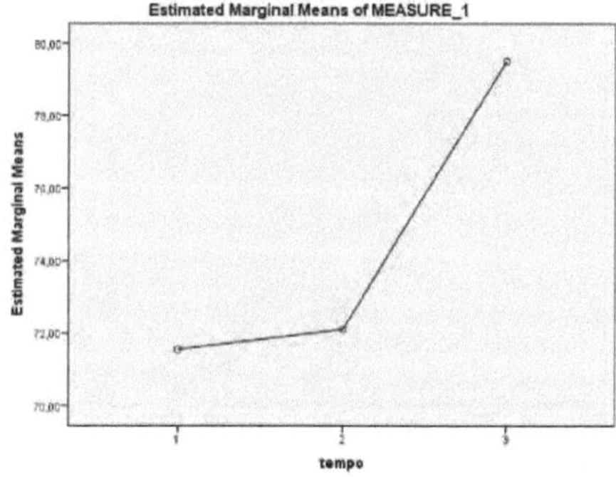

Figura 7 - General State of Health - SF-36, Passo Fundo, 2015

Figure 8 shows a significant variation in the vitality domain over time (p<0.001). There was a non-statistically significant reduction in the score post-surgery compared to baseline, mean difference 0.6 (95%CI -5.4 - 6.7, p=0.833), a statistically significant increase in the three-month follow-up compared to post-surgery, mean difference 16.4 (95%CI 10.5 - 22.2, p<0.001), also significantly higher than the baseline score, mean difference 15.7 (95%CI 9.9 - 21.5, p<0.001).

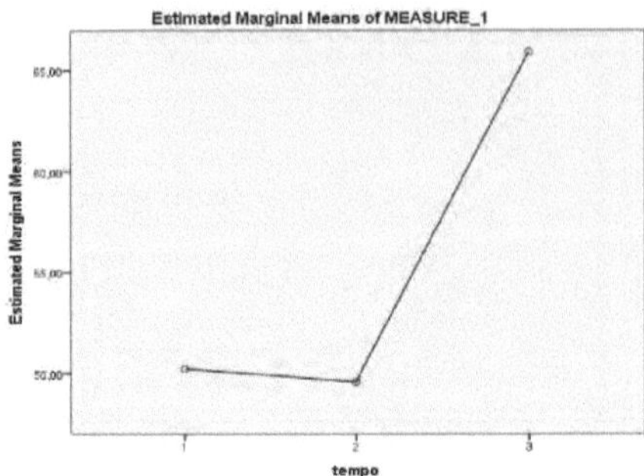

Figura 8 - Vitality - SF-36, Passo Fundo, 2015

There was a significant variation in the social aspects of time domain (p<0.001). There was a non-statistically significant reduction in the score post-surgery compared to baseline, mean difference 2.5 (95%CI -5.4 - 10.4, p=0.531), a statistically significant increase at three months follow-up compared to post-surgery, mean difference 21.1 (95%CI 13.6 - 28.6, p<0.001), also significantly higher than the baseline score, mean difference 18.6 (95%CI 10.6 - 26.5, p<0.001). (Figure 9).

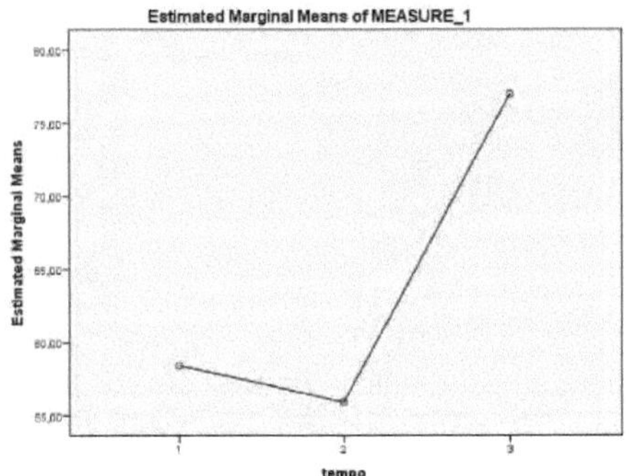

Figura 9 - Social Aspects - SF-36, Passo Fundo, 2015

Figure 10 shows a significant variation in the limitation by emotional aspects domain over time (p<0.001). Despite a significant reduction in the post-surgery score compared to baseline, mean difference 11.4 (95% CI 1.1 - 21.8, p=0.031), there was a recovery at the three-month follow-up, mean difference compared to post-surgery 39.1 (95% CI 27.3 - 50.8, p<0.001), reaching higher values than baseline, mean difference 27.6 (95% CI 15.0 - 40.2, p<0.001).

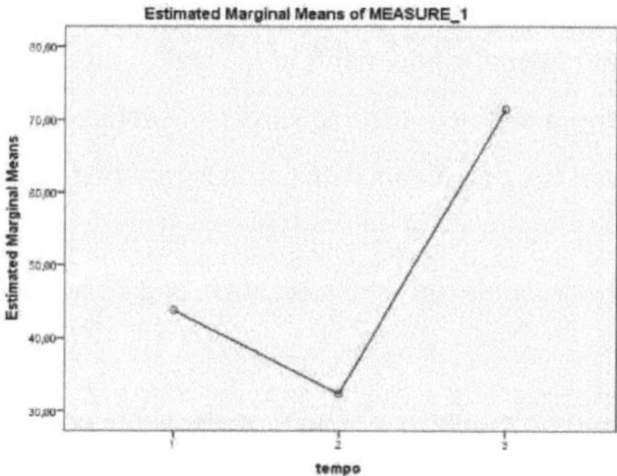

Figura 10 - Emotional Aspects - SF-36, Passo Fundo, 2015

Figure 11 shows a significant variation in the mental health domain over time (p<0.001). There was a non-statistically significant increase in the score post-surgery compared to baseline, mean difference 3.3 (95%CI -2.7 - 9.2, p=0.282), a statistically significant increase at three months follow-up compared to post-surgery, mean difference 9.2 (95%CI 4.5 - 13.9, p<0.001), also significantly higher than the baseline score, mean difference 12.5 (95%CI 7.0 - 17.9, p=0.001).

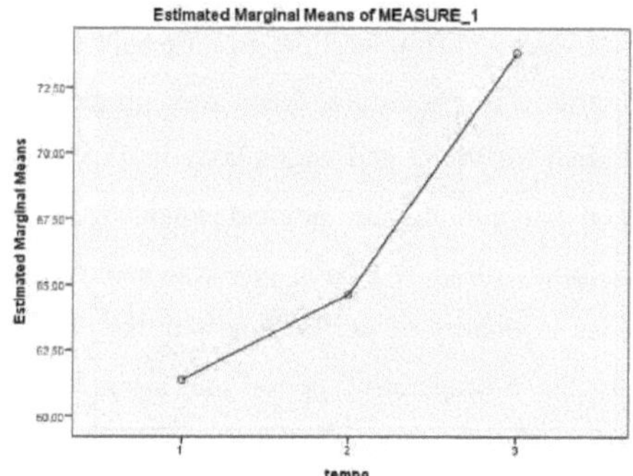

Figura 11 - Mental Health - SF-36, Passo Fundo, 2015

4. 4Discussion

This study assessed the quality of life of patients undergoing cardiac surgery at three different points in time: preoperative, postoperative and three-month follow-up, using the SF-36 instrument. This assessment tool analyzes data on physical health (functional capacity, physical aspects, pain and general state of health) and mental health (vitality, social aspect, emotional aspect and mental health) and is used to measure possible changes in quality of life as a result of certain medical interventions.

This study found an improvement in all the domains of the physical and mental components after three months of cardiac surgery, corroborating the study by Takiuti et al. (2007) which assessed quality of life after angioplasty, clinical treatment or coronary artery bypass grafting and found an improvement in all the domains, both in the physical and mental components at the end of the study, and this improvement was more marked in patients who underwent cardiac surgery. Another study carried out by Favarato et al (2006) assessed the quality of life of patients with coronary artery disease (CAD) who underwent one of three treatments: clinical, surgical or αngioplasty, at three different points in time, and showed that the changes in results between the initial phase, at six and 12 months were significant in the physical and mental dimensions.

Bahramnezhad et al. (2015) carried out a study evaluating the quality of life in patients undergoing percutaneous coronary angioplasty, with evaluations carried out before the procedure, three, six and 12 months after the procedure. Their results showed that there was no significant difference in quality of life before the procedure and three months after, but there was an improvement in quality of life at six months and 12 months post-procedure. This lack of improvement in quality of life three months after angioplasty, found in the above study, contradicts the results found in the present study, where there was an improvement in quality of life in the evaluation carried out three months after heart surgery.

In order to compare the quality of life of patients who underwent different treatments, the study revealed that patients who underwent coronary artery bypass grafting had the worst results in the initial assessment, but at six and twelve months after the procedure there was progressive improvement, surpassing patients who underwent clinical treatment and angioplasty in almost all dimensions of the SF-36. Therefore, it can be considered that, although the surgical patients were the most compromised in their quality of life from the point of view of the physical and mental components, the surgery provided a significant increase in quality of life, in line with the present study, which found a worsening of quality of life in the postoperative period and a significant improvement in quality of life three months after the procedure (FAVARATO et al., 2006).

Quality of life was assessed in patients undergoing on-pump and off-pump coronary artery bypass grafting. Significant changes were observed in both the physical and mental components. In the physical component, patients achieved significant improvement in all domains. This same condition was observed in the mental component. However, when we compared these results between the two forms of therapy (on-pump and off-pump CABG), these differences were not perceptible (NOGUEIRA et al., 2008).

Gois, Dantas and Torrati (2009) assessed health-related quality of life before and six months after the coronary artery bypass grafting procedure. They found that, preoperatively, four components of the SF-36 had lower scores, showing greater impairment in the following components: physical aspects, emotional aspects, functional capacity and pain. Six months after the surgical procedure, there was a statistically significant improvement in the evaluation of the eight components of the SF-36. The physical aspects and emotional aspects were the components that showed the best evaluation among the others. These data are in line with the results found in this study.

In the study carried out by Abelha et al. (2010), in which quality of life and mortality were assessed in patients with severe cardiac events in the postoperative period in general, 31% of the patients declared that their general health was better on the day they completed the SF-36 questionnaire than twelve months earlier, while 31% considered their health to be worse. The results of the SF-36 questionnaire of all patients who developed serious cardiac events were worse in all domains except body pain and mental health. However, this was a limitation of the study, as they didn't administer the SF-36 questionnaire before surgery, so it wasn't possible to compare the quality of life of the individuals before and after surgery.

In the present study, there was a significant decrease in the pain domain over time ($p<0.001$), corroborating Choinière et al. (2014) who carried out a two-year prospective multicenter study evaluating the prevalence and risk factors for persistent non-anginal pain after cardiac surgery. In their study, they showed that the prevalence of postoperative pain decreased significantly over time, 40.1% at three months, 22.1% at six months, 16.5% at 12 months and 9.5% at 24 months.

4.5 Conclusion

The study showed that patients undergoing cardiac surgery have an improved quality of life three months after the procedure. All domains, both physical and mental health components, showed significantly positive results.

4.6 References

ABELHA, F. J. et al. Evaluation of Quality of Life and Mortality in Patients with Severe Cardiac Events in the Postoperative Period. **Rev Bras Anestesiol**, v. 60, n. 3, p. 268-284, 2010.

AIKAWA, P. et al. Cardiac rehabilitation in patients undergoing coronary artery bypass graft surgery. **Rev Bras Med Esporte**, v. 20, n. 1, p. 55-58, 2014.

ALEXANDER, H. .; GLASSMAN, M. D. .; SHAPIRO, P. A. Depression and the Course of Coronary Artery Disease. **Am J Psychiatry**, v. 155, n. 1, p. 4-11, 1998.

ALMEIDA, F. F. et al. Predictors of Hospital Mortality and Severe Per-Operative Complications in Myocardial Revascularization Surgery. **Arq Bras Cardiol**, v. 80, n. nº 1, p. 41-50, 2003.

ANDERSON, A. J. P. G. et al. Predictors of mortality in patients over 70 years of age undergoing coronary artery bypass grafting or valve replacement with cardiopulmonary bypass. **Rev Bras Cir Cardiovasc**, v. 26, n. 1, p. 69-75, 2011.

BAHRAMNEZHAD, F. et al. Quality of Life in Patients Undergoing Percutaneous Transluminal Coronary Angioplasty (PTCA). **Global journal of health science**, v. 7, n. 5, p. 246-50, jan. 2015.

BATTAGIN, A. M.; CANINEU, P. R. Evaluation of functional capacity and depressive symptoms after cardiac surgery. **O Mundo da Saùde Sao Paulo**, v. 32, n. 2, p. 189-197, 2008.

BIANCO, A. C. M. et al. Prospective Risk Analysis in Patients Undergoing Myocardial Revascularization Surgery. **Arquivos Brasileiros de Cardiologia**, v. 85, n. 4, p. 254-261, 2005.

CARNEIRO, A. F. et al. Evaluation of Anxiety and Depression in the Preoperative Period in Patients Undergoing Invasive Cardiac Procedures *. **Rev Bras Anestesiol**, v. 59, n. 4, p. 431-438, 2009.

CARVALHO, A. L. DE O. **Quality of life after coronary artery bypass grafting, angioplasty or clinical treatment: 10-year follow-up**. [s.l.] University of Sao Paulo, 2013.

CARVALHO, L. D. P.; MEMEDE, M. V.; ARAÙJO, M. DOS R. O. Conhecimento de pacientes sobre o processo de auto-cuidado em pós-operatório de cirurgia cardiaca. **Cad. Pesq.**, v. 18, p. 18-25, 2011.

CHAUDHURY, S.; SRIVASTAVA, K. Relation of Depression , Anxiety , and Quality of Life with Outcome after Percutaneous Transluminal Coronary Angioplasty. **The Scientific World Journal**, v. 2013, 2013.

CHEIK, N. C. et al. Effects of physical exercise and physical activity on depression and anxiety in elderly individuals. **R. Bras. Ci. e Mov.**, v. 11, n. 3, p. 45-52, 2003.

CHOINIÈRE, M. et al. Prevalence of and risk factors for persistent postoperative nonangial pain after cardiac surgery : a 2-year prospective multicenter study. **CMAJ**, v. 186, n. 7, p. 213-23, 2014.

CICONELLI, R. M. et al. Translation into Portuguese and validation of the SF-36 (Brazil SF-36) generic quality of life assessment questionnaire. **Rev Bras Reumatol**, v. 39, n. 3, p. 143-50, 1999.

CSERÉP, Z. et al. Self-rated health is associated with the length of stay at the intensive care unit and hospital following cardiac surgery. v. 14, n. 171, p. 1-9, 2014.

CUSTÓDIO, F. M.; GASPARINO, R. C. Quality of Life of Patients in the Postoperative Cardiac Surgery Phase. **Reme: Revista Mineira de Enfermagem**, v. 17, n. 1, p. 130-134, 2013.

DANTAS, R. A. S.; AGUILLAR, O. M. Problems in the recovery of patients submitted to myocardial revascularization surgery: follow-up by nurses during the first month after hospital discharge. **Rev Latino-am Enfermagem**, v. 9, n. 6, p. 31-36, 2001.

DAYAN, V.; RICCA, R. Cardiac rehabilitation after coronary artery bypass grafting. v. 84, n. 4, p. 286-292, 2014.

FAVARATO, M. E. C. DE S. et al. Quality of life in patients with coronary artery disease: comparison between genders. **Rev Assoc Med Bras**, v. 52, n. 4, p. 23641, 2006.

FERREIRA, L. B.; VEIGAS, M. O. **Epidemiological profile of patients undergoing cardiac surgery at the Santa Genoveva Hospital in Goiânia**. [s.l.] Universidade Católiga de Goiàs, 2004.

FURUYA, R. K. et al. Anxiety and depression among men and women who underwent percutaneous coronary intervention. **Rev da Esc de Enferm USP**, v. 47, n. 6, p. 1333-7, dec. 2013.

GALDEANO, L. E. et al. Nursing diagnoses in the perioperative period of cardiac surgery. **Rev Esc Enferm USP**, v. 40, n. 1, p. 26-33, 2006.

GARBOSSA, A. et al. Effects of physiotherapeutic guidance on anxiety in patients undergoing coronary artery bypass graft surgery. **Rev Bras Cardiovasc**, v. 24, n. 3, p. 359-366, 2009.

GOIS, C. F. L. **Health-related quality of life, depression and sense of coherence of patients before and six months after coronary artery bypass grafting**. [s.l.] University of São Paulo, 2009.

GOIS, C. F. L.; DANTAS, R. A. S.; TORRATI, F. G. Health-related quality of life before and six months after coronary artery bypass grafting. **Rev Gaûcha Enferm**, v. 30, n. 4, p. 700-707, 2009.

HAWKES, A. L. et al. Outcomes of coronary artery bypass graft surgery. **Vascular Health and Risk Management**, v. 2, n. 4, p. 477-484, 2006.

KOERICH, C. et al. Myocardial revascularization: strategies for coping with the disease and the surgical process. **Acta Paul Enferm**, v. 26, n. 1, p. 8-13, 2013.

LESPÉRANCE; FRASURE-SMITH. Depression in patients with cardiac disease : a practical review. **Journal of Psychosomatic Research**, v. 48, p. 379-391, 2000.

LIMA, F. E. T. et al. Protocol for nursing consultations with patients after coronary artery bypass grafting: influence on anxiety and depression. **Rev Latino-am Enfermagem**, v. 18, n. 3, p. 35-41, 2010.

LIMA, M. S. et al. Depression in clinical and surgical patients admitted to a general hospital. **Arq Ciênc Saùde**, v. 12, n. 2, p. 63-66, 2005.

LOURES, D. R. DA R. L. et al. Cardiac surgery in the elderly. **Rev Bras Cir Cardiovasc**, v. 15, n. 1, p. 1-5, 2000.

MARCOLINO, J. A. M. et al. Measurement of anxiety and depression in preoperative patients. Comparative study. **Rev Bras Anestesiol**, v. 57, n. 2, p. 157166, 2007.

MESQUITA, E. T. et al. Quality of Care Indicators in Revascularization Surgery. **Arq Bras Cardiol**, v. 90, n. 5, p. 350-354, 2008.

MINAYO, M. C. DE S.; HARTZ, Z. M. DE A.; BUSS, P. M. Qualidade de vida e saù: um debate necessàrio. **Ciências & Saùde Coletiva**, v. 5, n. 1, p. 7-18, 2000.

MOERMAN, N. et al. The Amsterdam Preoperative Anxiety and Information Scale (APAIS). **Anesth Analg**, v. 82, p. 445-51, 1996.

MONTEIRO, R. et al. Quality of life in focus. **Rev Bras Cardiovasc**, v. 25, n. 4, p. 568-574, 2010.

MORIEL, G. et al. Quality of Life in Patients with Severe and Stable Coronary Atherosclerotic Disease. **Arq Bras Cardiol**, v. 95, n. 6, p. 691-697, 2010.

NOGUEIRA, C. R. S. R. . et al. Quality of Life after Coronary Artery Bypass Grafting with and without Cardiopulmonary Bypass. **Arq Bras Cardiol**, v. 91, n. 4, p. 238-244, 2008.

NOVAES, M. A. F. P.; ROMANO, B. W.; LAGE, S. G. Hospitalization in the ICU. Variables that Interfere in the Emotional Response. **Arq Bras Cardiol**, v. 67, n. 2, p. 99102, 1996.

NOVATO, T. DE S.; GROSSI, S. A. A.; KIMURA, M. Quality of life instrument for young people with diabetes. **Rev Gaûcha Enferm**, v. 28, n. 4, p. 512-519, 2007.

OLIVEIRA, S. K. P. et al. Nursing diagnosis present in adult patients in the postoperative of cardiac surgery. **Rev Enferm UFPI**, v. 1, n. 2, p. 95-100, 2012.

PIGNAY-DEMARIA, V. et al. Depression and Anxiety and Outcomes of Coronary Artery Bypass Surgery. **Ann Thorac Surg**, v. 75, p. 314-21, 2003.

PINTON, F. A. et al. Depression as a risk factor for immediate and late morbidity after coronary artery bypass grafting. **Braz J Cardiovasc Surg**, v. 21, n. 1, p. 68-74, 2006.

PLOTEK, W. et al. Emotional processes in patients undergoing coronary artery bypass graft surgeries with extracorporeal circulation in view of selected indicators of the inflammatory condition. **Med Sci Monit**, v. 21, p. 105-17, jan. 2015.

QUINTANA, J. F.; KALIL, R. A. K. Cardiac surgery: psychological manifestations of the patient in the pre- and postoperative period. **Psicologia Hospitalar**, v. 10, n. 2, p. 16-32, 2012.

ROGERS, W. J. et al. Ten-year follow-up of quality of life in patients randomized to receive medical therapy or coronary artery bypass graft surgery. The Coronary Artery Surgery Study (CASS). **Circulation**, v. 82, n. 5, p. 1647-1658, 1 nov. 1990.

SHERWOOD, A. et al. Impaired endothelial function in coronary heart disease patients with depressive symptomatology. **Journal of the American College of Cardiology**, v. 46, n. 4, p. 656-9, Aug. 16, 2005.

TAKIUTI, M. E. et al. Quality of life after coronary artery bypass grafting, angioplasty or clinical treatment. **Arq Bras Cardiol**, v. 88, n. 5, p. 537-544, 2007.

TANAJURA, D. et al. Prevalence of depression in different groups of inpatients at the University Hospital of Bahia , Brazil. **Rev Bras Psiquiatr**, v. 24, n. 4, p. 182185, 2002.

TIMBERLAKE, N. et al. Incidence and patterns of depression following coronary artery bypass graft surgery. **Journal of Psychosomatic Research**, v. 43, n. 2, p. 197-207, 1997.

TONIAL, R.; MOREIRA, D. M. Clinical-epidemiological profile of patients undergoing coronary artery bypass grafting at the Santa Catarina Institute of Cardiology, Sao José - SC. **Arquivos Catarineses de Medicina**, v. 40, n. 4, p. 42-46, 2011.

TORRATI, F. G. **Anxiety, depression, sense of coherence and stressors in the pre- and postoperative periods of cardiac surgery**. [s.l.] University of Sao Paulo, 2009.

VARGAS, T. V. P.; DANTAS, R. A. S.; GOIS, C. F. L. The self-esteem of individuals who have undergone coronary artery bypass graft surgery. **Rev Esc Enferm USP**, v. 39, n. 1, p. 20-27, 2005.

VARGAS, T. V. P.; MAIA, E. M.; DANTAS, R. A. S. Sentiments of patients in the preoperative period of cardiac surgery. **Rev Latino-am Enfermagem**, v. 14, n. 3, p. 1-6, 2006.

VILA, V. DA S. C.; ROSSI, L. A.; COSTA, M. C. S. Experience of heart disease among adults undergoing coronary artery bypass grafting. **Rev Saùde Pùblica**, v. 42, n. 4, 2008.

WINKELMANN, E. R.; MANFROI, W. C. Quality of life in cardiology. **Rev HCPA**, v. 28, n. 1, p. 49-53, 2008.

5 FINAL CONSIDERATIONS

The daily care of patients undergoing cardiac surgery has given us an insight into the anxieties, feelings and fears these patients have. Based on this experience and due to the great relevance of this topic today, given the increasing indication for and performance of heart surgery, the need arose to evaluate the emotional aspect of patients undergoing these procedures, as well as the relationship between these aspects and the prognosis and quality of life of these individuals.

So we carried out this study, which allowed us to get to know patients undergoing heart surgery even more closely. In this study, we had the opportunity to assess the patients on three different occasions, each of which allowed us to deepen our relationship with the patients.

This study highlighted the need of patients undergoing heart surgery for mental and emotional health, which is often neglected by health professionals. Symptoms suggestive of depression and anxiety were present at significant levels in these patients, which indicates the need for more patient-centered care as a whole, including an adequate emotional approach by all team members, and not just the performance of the specific techniques of each professional.

It is believed that this research was highly relevant to the development of the various professionals involved in the care of these patients, bringing more quality and knowledge to the members of the multiprofessional teams of the hospitals involved, culminating in better patient care. In addition, the results of this study may contribute to improving care in institutions in general that did not take part in the study.

Carrying out this research has been extremely rewarding for me personally, as it has enabled me to acquire not only knowledge but also numerous interpersonal experiences, making it possible to understand how much such a delicate procedure as heart surgery affects the lives of patients and their families. In addition, this research has promoted great professional growth, providing data that will enable us to offer more qualified care to patients undergoing cardiac surgery.

REFERENCES

ABELHA, F. J. et al. Evaluation of Quality of Life and Mortality in Patients with Severe Cardiac Events in the Postoperative Period. **Rev Bras Anestesiol**, v. 60, n. 3, p. 268-284, 2010.

AIKAWA, P. et al. Cardiac rehabilitation in patients undergoing coronary artery bypass graft surgery. **Rev Bras Med Esporte**, v. 20, n. 1, p. 55-58, 2014.

ALEXANDER, H. .; GLASSMAN, M. D. .; SHAPIRO, P. A. Depression and the Course of Coronary Artery Disease. **Am J Psychiatry**, v. 155, n. 1, p. 4-11, 1998.

ALMEIDA, F. F. et al. Predictors of Hospital Mortality and Severe Per-Operative Complications in Myocardial Revascularization Surgery. **Arq Bras Cardiol**, v. 80, n. nº 1, p. 41-50, 2003.

ANDERSON, A. J. P. G. et al. Predictors of mortality in patients over 70 years of age undergoing coronary artery bypass grafting or valve replacement with cardiopulmonary bypass. **Rev Bras Cir Cardiovasc**, v. 26, n. 1, p. 69-75, 2011.

BAHRAMNEZHAD, F. et al. Quality of Life in Patients Undergoing Percutaneous Transluminal Coronary Angioplasty (PTCA). **Global journal of health science**, v. 7, n. 5, p. 246-50, jan. 2015.

BATTAGIN, A. M.; CANINEU, P. R. Evaluation of functional capacity and depressive symptoms after cardiac surgery. **O Mundo da Saùde Sao Paulo**, v. 32, n. 2, p. 189-197, 2008.

BIANCO, A. C. M. et al. Prospective Risk Analysis in Patients Undergoing Myocardial Revascularization Surgery. **Arquivos Brasileiros de Cardiologia**, v. 85, n. 4, p. 254-261, 2005.

CARNEIRO, A. F. et al. Evaluation of Anxiety and Depression in the Preoperative Period in Patients Undergoing Invasive Cardiac Procedures *. **Rev Bras Anestesiol**, v. 59, n. 4, p. 431-438, 2009.

CARVALHO, A. L. DE O. **Quality of life after coronary artery bypass grafting, angioplasty or clinical treatment: 10-year follow-up**. [s.l.] University of Sao Paulo, 2013.

CARVALHO, L. D. P.; MEMEDE, M. V.; ARAÙJO, M. DOS R. O. Conhecimento de pacientes sobre o processo de auto-cuidado em pós-operatório de cirurgia cardiaca. **Cad. Pesq.**, v. 18, p. 18-25, 2011.

CHAUDHURY, S.; SRIVASTAVA, K. Relation of Depression , Anxiety , and Quality of Life with Outcome after Percutaneous Transluminal Coronary Angioplasty. **The Scientific World Journal**, v. 2013, 2013.

CHEIK, N. C. et al. Effects of physical exercise and physical activity on depression and anxiety in elderly individuals. **R. Bras. Ci. e Mov.**, v. 11, n. 3, p. 45-52, 2003.

CHOINIÈRE, M. et al. Prevalence of and risk factors for persistent postoperative nonangial pain after cardiac surgery : a 2-year prospective multicenter study. **CMAJ**, v. 186, n. 7, p. 213-23, 2014.

CICONELLI, R. M. et al. Translation into Portuguese and validation of the SF-36 (Brazil SF-36) generic quality of life assessment questionnaire. **Rev Bras Reumatol**, v. 39, n. 3, p. 143-50, 1999.

CSERÉP, Z. et al. Self-rated health is associated with the length of stay at the intensive care unit and hospital following cardiac surgery. v. 14, n. 171, p. 1-9, 2014.

CUSTÓDIO, F. M.; GASPARINO, R. C. Quality of Life of Patients in the Postoperative Cardiac Surgery Phase. **Reme: Revista Mineira de Enfermagem**, v. 17, n. 1, p. 130-134, 2013.

DANTAS, R. A. S.; AGUILLAR, O. M. Problems in the recovery of patients submitted to myocardial revascularization surgery: follow-up by nurses during the first month after hospital discharge. **Rev Latino-am Enfermagem**, v. 9, n. 6, p. 31-36, 2001.

DAYAN, V.; RICCA, R. Cardiac rehabilitation after coronary artery bypass grafting. v. 84, n. 4, p. 286-292, 2014.

FAVARATO, M. E. C. DE S. et al. Quality of life in patients with coronary artery disease: comparison between genders. **Rev Assoc Med Bras**, v. 52, n. 4, p. 23641, 2006.

FERREIRA, L. B.; VEIGAS, M. O. **Epidemiological profile of patients undergoing cardiac surgery at the Santa Genoveva Hospital in Goiânia**. [s.l.] Universidade Católiga de Goiàs, 2004.

FURUYA, R. K. et al. Anxiety and depression among men and women who underwent percutaneous coronary intervention. **Rev da Esc de Enferm USP**, v. 47, n. 6, p. 1333-7, dec. 2013.

GALDEANO, L. E. et al. Nursing diagnoses in the perioperative period of cardiac surgery. **Rev Esc Enferm USP**, v. 40, n. 1, p. 26-33, 2006.

GARBOSSA, A. et al. Effects of physiotherapeutic guidance on anxiety in patients undergoing coronary artery bypass graft surgery. **Rev Bras Cardiovasc**, v. 24, n. 3, p. 359-366, 2009.

GOIS, C. F. L. **Health-related quality of life, depression and sense of coherence of patients before and six months after coronary artery bypass grafting**. [s.l.] University of Sao Paulo, 2009.

GOIS, C. F. L.; DANTAS, R. A. S.; TORRATI, F. G. Health-related quality of life before and six months after coronary artery bypass grafting. **Rev Gaûcha Enferm**, v. 30, n. 4, p. 700-707, 2009.

HAWKES, A. L. et al. Outcomes of coronary artery bypass graft surgery. **Vascular Health and Risk Management**, v. 2, n. 4, p. 477-484, 2006.

KOERICH, C. et al. Myocardial revascularization: strategies for coping with the disease and the surgical process. **Acta Paul Enferm**, v. 26, n. 1, p. 8-13, 2013.

LESPÉRANCE; FRASURE-SMITH. Depression in patients with cardiac disease : a practical review.

Journal of Psychosomatic Research, v. 48, p. 379-391, 2000.

LIMA, F. E. T. et al. Protocol for nursing consultations with patients after coronary artery bypass grafting: influence on anxiety and depression. **Rev Latino-am Enfermagem**, v. 18, n. 3, p. 35-41, 2010.

LIMA, M. S. et al. Depression in clinical and surgical patients admitted to a general hospital. **Arq Ciênc Saùde**, v. 12, n. 2, p. 63-66, 2005.

LOURES, D. R. DA R. L. et al. Cardiac surgery in the elderly. **Rev Bras Cir Cardiovasc**, v. 15, n. 1, p. 1-5, 2000.

MARCOLINO, J. A. M. et al. Measurement of anxiety and depression in preoperative patients. Comparative study. **Rev Bras Anestesiol**, v. 57, n. 2, p. 157166, 2007.

MESQUITA, E. T. et al. Quality of Care Indicators in Revascularization Surgery. **Arq Bras Cardiol**, v. 90, n. 5, p. 350-354, 2008.

MINAYO, M. C. DE S.; HARTZ, Z. M. DE A.; BUSS, P. M. Qualidade de vida e saù: um debate necessàrio. **Ciências & Saùde Coletiva**, v. 5, n. 1, p. 7-18, 2000.

MOERMAN, N. et al. The Amsterdam Preoperative Anxiety and Information Scale (APAIS). **Anesth Analg**, v. 82, p. 445-51, 1996.

MONTEIRO, R. et al. Quality of life in focus. **Rev Bras Cardiovasc**, v. 25, n. 4, p. 568-574, 2010.

MORIEL, G. et al. Quality of Life in Patients with Severe and Stable Coronary Atherosclerotic Disease. **Arq Bras Cardiol**, v. 95, n. 6, p. 691-697, 2010.

NOGUEIRA, C. R. S. R. . et al. Quality of Life after Myocardial Revascularization with and without Extracorporeal Circulation. **Arq Bras Cardiol**, v. 91, n. 4, p. 238-244, 2008.

NOVAES, M. A. F. P.; ROMANO, B. W.; LAGE, S. G. ICU Hospitalization. Variables that Interfere in the Emotional Response. **Arq Bras Cardiol**, v. 67, n. 2, p. 99102, 1996.

NOVATO, T. DE S.; GROSSI, S. A. A.; KIMURA, M. Quality of life instrument for young people with diabetes. **Rev Gaûcha Enferm**, v. 28, n. 4, p. 512-519, 2007.

OLIVEIRA, S. K. P. et al. Nursing diagnosis present in adult patients in the postoperative of cardiac surgery. **Rev Enferm UFPI**, v. 1, n. 2, p. 95-100, 2012.

PIGNAY-DEMARIA, V. et al. Depression and Anxiety and Outcomes of Coronary Artery Bypass Surgery. **Ann Thorac Surg**, v. 75, p. 314-21, 2003.

PINTON, F. A. et al. Depression as a risk factor for immediate and late morbidity after coronary artery bypass grafting. **Braz J Cardiovasc Surg**, v. 21, n. 1, p. 68-74, 2006.

PLOTEK, W. et al. Emotional processes in patients undergoing coronary artery bypass graft surgeries with extracorporeal circulation in view of selected indicators of the inflammatory condition. **Med Sci Monit**, v. 21, p. 105-17, jan. 2015.

QUINTANA, J. F.; KALIL, R. A. K. Cardiac surgery: psychological manifestations of the patient in the pre- and postoperative period. **Psicologia Hospitalar**, v. 10, n. 2, p. 16-32, 2012.

ROGERS, W. J. et al. Ten-year follow-up of quality of life in patients randomized to receive medical therapy or coronary artery bypass graft surgery. The Coronary Artery Surgery Study (CASS). **Circulation**, v. 82, n. 5, p. 1647-1658, 1 nov. 1990.

SHERWOOD, A. et al. Impaired endothelial function in coronary heart disease patients with depressive symptomatology. **Journal of the American College of Cardiology**, v. 46, n. 4, p. 656-9, Aug. 16, 2005.

TAKIUTI, M. E. et al. Quality of life after coronary artery bypass grafting, angioplasty or clinical treatment. **Arq Bras Cardiol**, v. 88, n. 5, p. 537-544, 2007.

TANAJURA, D. et al. Prevalence of depression in different groups of inpatients at the University Hospital of Bahia , Brazil. **Rev Bras Psiquiatr**, v. 24, n. 4, p. 182185, 2002.

TIMBERLAKE, N. et al. Incidence and patterns of depression following coronary artery bypass graft surgery. **Journal of Psychosomatic Research**, v. 43, n. 2, p. 197-207, 1997.

TONIAL, R.; MOREIRA, D. M. Clinical-epidemiological profile of patients undergoing coronary artery bypass grafting at the Santa Catarina Institute of Cardiology, Sao José - SC. **Arquivos Catarineses de Medicina**, v. 40, n. 4, p. 42-46, 2011.

TORRATI, F. G. **Anxiety, depression, sense of coherence and stressors in the pre- and postoperative periods of cardiac surgery**. [s.l.] University of Sao Paulo, 2009.

VARGAS, T. V. P.; DANTAS, R. A. S.; GOIS, C. F. L. The self-esteem of individuals who have undergone coronary artery bypass graft surgery. **Rev Esc Enferm USP**, v. 39, n. 1, p. 20-27, 2005.

VARGAS, T. V. P.; MAIA, E. M.; DANTAS, R. A. S. Sentiments of patients in the preoperative period of cardiac surgery. **Rev Latino-am Enfermagem**, v. 14, n. 3, p. 1-6, 2006.

VILA, V. DA S. C.; ROSSI, L. A.; COSTA, M. C. S. Experience of heart disease among adults undergoing coronary artery bypass grafting. **Rev Saùde Pùblica**, v. 42, n. 4, 2008.

WINKELMANN, E. R.; MANFROI, W. C. Quality of life in cardiology. **Rev HCPA**, v. 28, n. 1, p. 49-53, 2008.

ANNEXES

Annex A. Authorization from the Research Management Center (CGP) and the Research and Postgraduate Commission (CPPG) - HSVP

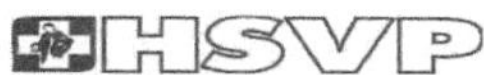

HOSPITAL SÃO VICENTE DE PAULO

Centro de Gerenciamento em Pesquisas (CGP- HSVP)

Comissão de Pesquisas e Pós-Graduação (CPPG)

Passo Fundo, 15 de janeiro de 2015.

Parecer

Autor(a): **Débora D'Agostini Jorge Lisboa.**

Orientador (a): Dra Eliane Lucia Colussi.

Responsável no HSVP: Dr. Luis Sérgio de Moura Fragomeni.

Caros Pesquisadores

A Comissão de Pesquisas e Pós-Graduação do Hospital São Vicente de Paulo analisou seu projeto de pesquisa intitulado: **"ANSIEDADE E SINTOMAS DEPRESSIVOS EM ADULTOS E IDOSOS SUBMETIDOS À CIRURGIA CARDÍACA PARA REVASCULARIZAÇÃO DO MIOCÁRDIO E/OU SUBSTITUIÇÃO VALVAR"** e **aprovou** o estudo, salientando que esse pode ser iniciado a partir dessa data.

Queremos lembrar a necessidade de o pesquisador manter o Centro de Gerenciamento (CGP-HSVP) atualizado, sobre o desenvolvimento científico dentro do Hospital, informando sobre a aprovação na Plataforma Brasil e incluindo o HSVP como Instituição co-participante na folha de rosto do CONEP, informando também sobre as publicações ou apresentações dos resultados desta pesquisa (relatórios parciais e finais deverão ser encaminhados a este setor).

A comissão agradece a iniciativa em pesquisar no Hospital Ensino São Vicente de Paulo, deseja um ótimo trabalho aos pesquisadores lembrando que sejam cumpridas as normas regulamentares do HSVP (a pesquisa não deve produzir riscos aos pacientes e ao Hospital).

Atenciosamente,

Dr. Hugo Lisboa
Coordenador CPPG-HSVP

Centro de Gerenciamento de Pesquisas (CGP-HSVP)

Valéria Sumye Milani
CPPG – HSVP

da Associação Hospitalar Beneficente São Vicente de Paulo (Entidade de Fins Filantrópicos)
Rua Teixeira Soares, 808 – Tel.: (0**54) 3316.4000 – Fax.: (0**54) 3316.4015 – CEP: 99.010-080 – PASSO FUNDO - RS

Annex B. Opinion of the Research Ethics Committee (CEP)

UNIVERSIDADE DE PASSO FUNDO/ PRÓ-REITORIA DE PESQUISA E PÓS-

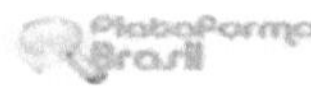

PARECER CONSUBSTANCIADO DO CEP

DADOS DO PROJETO DE PESQUISA

Título da Pesquisa: Ansiedade e sintomas depressivos em adultos e idosos submetidos à cirurgia cardíaca

Pesquisador: Débora D'Agostini Jorge Lisboa
Área Temática:
Versão: 2
CAAE: 41816414.1.0000.5342
Instituição Proponente: UNIVERSIDADE DE PASSO FUNDO
Patrocinador Principal: Financiamento Próprio

DADOS DO PARECER

Número do Parecer: 1.029.446
Data da Relatoria: 27/04/2015

Apresentação do Projeto:
As doenças cardíacas crônicas constituem um grupo de patologias altamente prevalentes no mundo todo, especialmente relacionadas com o fenômeno de envelhecimento populacional observado nos últimos anos. Dentre as modalidades terapêuticas disponíveis para estas enfermidades, encontramos a cirurgia cardíaca, um procedimento invasivo de alto risco, que envolve fatores complexos como manipulação cardíaca e circulação extracorpórea, que na grande maioria das vezes são acompanhados de complicações físicas e psicológicas. A necessidade de uma cirurgia cardíaca normalmente vem acompanhada de fragilização e medo por parte dos pacientes, assim, torna-se comum o surgimento ou exacerbação de sintomas de ansiedade e depressão nestes pacientes. Estudos comprovam que a ansiedade e a depressão podem

Endereço: BR 285- Km 292 Campus I - Centro Administrativo
Bairro: Divisão de Pesquisa / São José **CEP:** 99.052-900
UF: RS **Município:** PASSO FUNDO
Telefone: (54)3316-8157 **E-mail:** cep@upf.br

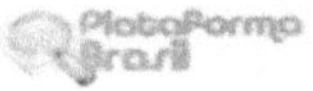

aumentar a morbimortalidade pós-operatória e alterar a qualidade da vida destes pacientes submetidos a cirurgia cardíaca. O presente estudo objetiva avaliar a presença de sintomas sugestivos de depressão e ansiedade em pacientes adultos e idosos em período anterior e posterior a cirurgia cardíaca para revascularização do miocárdio e substituição valvar

Objetivo da Pesquisa:
Avaliar a presença de sintomas sugestivos de depressão e ansiedade em pacientes adultos e idosos em período anterior e posterior a cirurgia cardíaca para revascularização do miocárdio e substituição valvar.

Avaliação dos Riscos e Benefícios:
De acordo com as pesquisadoras, o benefício da pesquisa será entender melhor a relação entre os sintomas de ansiedade e depressão e cirurgia cardíaca, e o efeito da cirurgia cardíaca na qualidade de vida dos pacientes.

Comentários e Considerações sobre a Pesquisa:
Estudo de coorte prospectivo não controlado com adultos e idosos submetidos à cirurgia cardíaca para revascularização do miocárdio e substituição valvar. O estudo será realizado no Hospital da Cidade de Passo Fundo e no Hospital São Vicente de Paulo de Passo Fundo. A coleta dos dados ocorrerá em três momentos distintos, pré-operatório, pós-operatório durante a internação hospitalar e após três meses do procedimento cirúrgico, por meio de Questionário Clínico Sóciodemográfico, Escala de Avaliação do Nível de Ansiedade e Depressão e Questionário de Qualidade de Vida SF-36.

Considerações sobre os Termos de apresentação obrigatória:
Os direitos fundamentais do(s) participante(s) foi(ram) garantido(s) no projeto e no TCLE. O protocolo foi instruído e apresentado de maneira completa e adequada. Os compromissos do (a) pesquisador (a) e das instituições envolvidas estavam presentes. O projeto foi considerado claro em seus aspectos científicos, metodológicos e éticos.

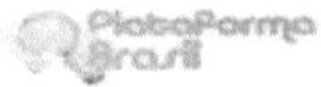

Recomendações:

Após o término da pesquisa, o CEP UPF solicita:

a) A devolução dos resultados do estudo ao(s) sujeito(s) da pesquisa ou a instituição que forneceu os dados;

b) Enviar o relatório final da pesquisa, pela plataforma, utilizando a opção, no final da página, "Enviar Notificação" + relatório final.

Conclusões ou Pendências e Lista de Inadequações:

Diante do exposto, este Comitê, de acordo com as atribuições definidas na Resolução n. 466/12, do Conselho Nacional da Saúde, Ministério da Saúde, Brasil, manifesta-se pela aprovação do projeto de pesquisa na forma como foi proposto.

Além do mais, o CEP poderá, a qualquer momento, acompanhar o andamento da pesquisa, de acordo com a Res. 466/12.

Situação do Parecer:

Aprovado

Necessita Apreciação da CONEP:

Não

Considerações Finais a critério do CEP:

Endereço: BR 285- Km 292 Campus I - Centro Administrativo
Bairro: Divisão de Pesquisa / São José **CEP:** 99.052-900
UF: RS **Município:** PASSO FUNDO
Telefone: (54)3316-8157 **E-mail:** cep@upf.br

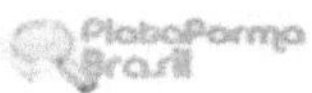

PASSO FUNDO, 20 de Abril de 2015

Assinado por:
Nadir Antonio Pichler
(Coordenador)

Endereço: BR 285- Km 292 Campus I - Centro Administrativo
Bairro: Divisão de Pesquisa / São José **CEP:** 99.052-900
UF: RS **Município:** PASSO FUNDO
Telefone: (54)3316-8157 **E-mail:** cep@upf.br

Annex C. Authorization from Passo Fundo City Hospital - HC

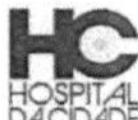

Rua Tiradentes, 295 – Passo Fundo/RS.
Cep 99010-260 – E-mail coreme@hcpf.com.br
Tel. (54) 2103 3333 – CNPJ: 92.030.543/0001-70

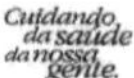

Passo Fundo, 30 de abril de 2015.

AUTORIZAÇÃO

Autorizo, no Hospital da Cidade de Passo Fundo, a realização da pesquisa **"ANSIEDADE E SINTOMAS DEPRESSIVOS EM ADULTOS E IDOSOS SUBMETIDOS À CIRURGIA CARDÍACA"** tendo como pesquisadora responsáve DÉBORA D'AGOSTINI JORGE LISBOA, do Curso de Fisioterapia da Universidade de Passo Fundo.

Dionísio Adelcir Balvedi
Membro da Junta Administrativa
Hospital da Cidade de Passo Fundo

APPENDICES

Appendix A. Informed Consent Form (ICF)

UPF University of Passo Fundo

Faculty of Physical Education and Physiotherapy

Postgraduate Program in Human Ageing

TERM OF FREE AND INFORMED CONSENT (TCLE)

Dear Sir or Madam

You are being invited to take part in a research project entitled "Anxiety and depressive symptoms in adults and elderly people undergoing heart surgery". The study is being carried out by me, Débora D'Agostini Jorge Lisboa, a student on the *stricto sensu* Postgraduate Program in Human Ageing at the University of Passo Fundo - UPF, under the supervision of Professor Eliane Lucia Colussi.

The aim of this study is to assess the presence of symptoms suggestive of depression and anxiety in adult and elderly patients before and after heart surgery. You will take part in the study by answering questions about your state of health, how you have been feeling recently and questions about your quality of life. There will be three meetings: phase I - before surgery, phase II - after surgery on discharge from hospital and phase III - three months after the procedure. At Hospital da Cidade de Passo Fundo, the phase III evaluation will take place in the cardiology outpatient clinic, located in the basement of the hospital, which is entered from Rua Uruguai. At the Sao Vicente de Paulo Hospital, the evaluation will take place in the specialties outpatient clinic, which is entered via Rua XV de Novembro. The evaluations at both hospitals will be carried out after the medical re-evaluation appointment, thus taking advantage of the patient's commute, so there will be no extra costs. The interviews in phases I, II and III will last approximately forty minutes each. Your participation does not imply any risk to your health or integrity, but if I identify any sign of discomfort, I undertake to interrupt the interview and refer you to professionals and/or specialized services in the field. As a benefit, at the end of the study you will be able to attend a lecture at the institution to hear the results of the study.

Your participation in this research is not compulsory and you can withdraw your consent at any time without any prejudice to your attendance at the institution or participation in the social group. I would like to make it clear that you will have answers to any questions or doubts about the research at any stage of the study. The results of this study will be disclosed for academic and scientific purposes and will not cause any damage or harm to you, with the guarantee of confidentiality and reliability of the data relating to your identification.

This form will be signed in two copies, one of which will remain with the researcher and the other with you. If you have any questions or clarifications regarding the research, you can contact the researcher on (54) 8126-4877, and the Research Ethics Committee of the University of Passo Fundo (Monday to Friday, from 8am to 12pm, and from 1.30pm to 5.30pm) on (54) 3316-8157.

In these terms and considering myself informed, I consent to participate in the proposed research, freely and spontaneously, without charge or any financial burden, safeguarding the authors of the project the intellectual property of the information generated and expressing agreement with the public disclosure of the results, signing this term in the place indicated below.

Thank you in advance for your cooperation

Passo Fundo, _______________ of ___ of 201

Participant's name

Participant's signature

Prof. Eliane Lucia Colussi Advisor

Researcher Débora D`Agostini Jorge Lisboa Master's student in Human Ageing

Note: This document, in accordance with Resolution No. 466/12 of the National Health Council, will be signed in two copies of equal content, one copy remaining in the possession of the participant and the other with the authors of the research.

Appendix B. Collection instrument I - Sociodemographic questionnaire

---

UPF University of Passo Fundo

Faculty of Physical Education and Physiotherapy

Postgraduate Program in Human Ageing

Clinical and sociodemographic characterization questionnaire

Personal Data

Name: ____

Address: ____

Phone: ( ) __________________ City/State: _______________________

Hospital: ______________________________

Sociodemographic data

Age Sex: ( ) female (_________) male

Marital status: ( ) single ( ) married ( ) divorced ( ) widowed ( )

other Education: ________________ in years City: ________________________

Lives: ( ) urban area ( )rural area Occupation:

( ) retired/ how long ___________________ Family income: _____________

Children: ( ) yes ( ) no How many _________Religion: ________________

Ethnicity: ( ) white ( ) brown ( ) Afro-descendant

Clinical Data

Type of surgery performed: ____

Date of surgery: ______________Basic pathology:__________________________

Cardiopulmonary bypass: ( ) yes ( ) no CPB time:____________________

Hospitalization date:DISCHARGE:ICU date:ICU DISCHARGE:

Length of illness:Length of hospitalization:

Previous depression: ( ) yes ( ) no In treatment: ( ) yes ( ) no

Reviewer: ____________________________________ Date: _________________

Appendix C. Collection Instrument II - HAD Scale

UPF University of Passo Fundo

Faculty of Physical Education and Physiotherapy

Postgraduate Program in Human Ageing

HAD Anxiety and Depression Scale

PERSONAL DATA			
NAME			
TEST GUIDELINES			
Mark with an "X" the alternative that best describes your answer to each question.			
1) I feel tense or contracted:			
( ) most of the time[3]	( ) much of the time[2]	( ) from time to time[1]	( ) never [0]
2. I still feel like I like the same things as before:			

( ) yes, the same as before [0]	( ) not as much as before [1]	( ) just a little [2]	( ) I can no longer take pleasure in anything [3]
3. I feel a kind of fear, as if something bad is going to happen			
( ) yes, very strongly [3]	( ) yes, but not so much strong [2]	( ) a bit, but that doesn't worry me [1]	( ) I don't feel anything like that[1]
4. I laugh and have fun when I see funny things			
( ) the same as before[0]	( ) currently a little less[1]	( ) currently much less[2]	( ) I can't do it anymore[3]
5. My head is full of worries			
( ) most of the time[3]	( ) much of the time[2]	( ) from time to time[1]	( ) rarely[0]
6. I feel happy			
( ) never[3]	( ) a few times[2]	( ) many times[1]	( ) most of the time[0]
7. I can sit at ease and feel relaxed:			
( ) yes, almost always[0]	( ) many times[1]	( ) a few times[2]	( ) never[3]
8. I'm slow to think and do things:			
( ) almost always[3]	( ) many times[2]	( ) a few times[1]	( ) never[0]
9. I get a bad feeling of fear, like a chill in my stomach or a tightness in my gut:			
( ) never[0]	( ) from time to time[1]	( ) many times[2]	( ) almost always[3]
10. I lost interest in taking care of my appearance:			
( ) completely[3]	( ) I'm not taking care of myself the way I used to I should[2]	( )maybe not as much as before[1]	( ) I take care of myself the same way as before[0]
11. I feel restless, as if I can't sit still anywhere:			
( ) yes, too much[3]	( ) a lot[2]	( ) a little[1]	( ) I don't feel that way[0]
12. I get excited waiting for the good things to come			
( ) in the same way as before[0]	( ) a a little less than before[1]	( ) much less than before[2]	( ) almost never[3]
13. Suddenly, I feel like I'm going to panic:			
( ) almost all the time[3]	( ) several times[2]	( ) from time to time[1]	( ) I didn't feel that[0]
14. I can feel pleasure when I watch a good TV or radio program or when I read something:			
( ) almost always[0]	( ) several times[1]	( ) a few times[2]	( ) almost never[3]
TEST RESULTS			
REMARKS:			
Anxiety: [ ] questions (1,3,5,7,9,11,13) **Depression: [ ] questions (2,4,6,8,10,12 and 14)**			

NAME RESPONSIBLE FOR ADMINISTERING THE TEST	I
DATE I	

Appendix D. Collection Instrument III - SF-36 Quality of Life Questionnaire

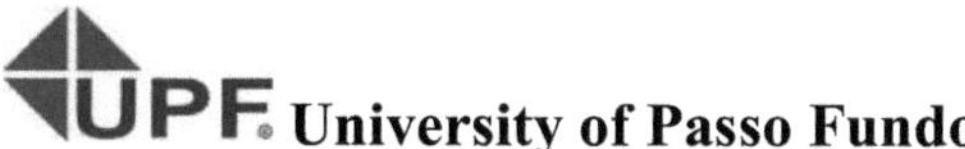

Faculty of Physical Education and Physiotherapy

Postgraduate Program in Human Ageing

Brazilian version of the Quality of Life Questionnaire-SF-36

Job function: ____

How long have you held this position? ______________________

Instructions: This survey asks you about your health. This information will keep us informed of how you feel and how well you are able to carry out activities of daily living. Please answer each question by marking the answer as indicated. If you are unsure how to answer, please try your best.

1- In general you would say your health is:

Excellent	Very good	Good	Bad	Very bad
1	2	3	4	5

2- Compared to a year ago, how would you rate your age in general now?

Much better	A Little Better	Almost the Same	A Little Worse	Much Worse
1	2	3	4	5

3- The following items are about activities that you could currently do during an average day. Due to your health, would you find it difficult to do these activities? If so, when?

Activities	Yes, it makes it very difficult	Yes, it's a bit difficult	No, it doesn't make it difficult at all
a) Rigorous activities, that demanding exertion, such as running, lifting heavy objects, participating in hard sports.	1	2	3
b) Moderate activities, such as moving a table, vacuuming, playing ball, sweeping the house.	1	2	3
c) Lifting or carrying supplies	1	2	3
d) Climbing several flights of stairs	1	2	3
e) Climbing a flight of stairs	1	2	3

f) Bowing, kneeling or bending down	1	2	3
g) Walking more than 1 kilometer	1	2	3
h) Walk several blocks	1	2	3
i) Walk a block	1	2	3
j) Bathing or dressing	1	2	3

4- During the last 4 weeks, have you had any of the following problems with your work or regular activity, as a consequence of your physical health?

	Yes	No
a) Have you reduced the amount of time you devote to your work or other activities?	1	2
b) Did you do fewer tasks than you would have liked?	1	2
c) You have been limited in your type of work or other activities.	1	2
d) Had difficulty doing your work or other activities (e.g. required extra effort).	1	2

5- During the last 4 weeks, have you had any of the following problems with your work or other regular daily activity as a result of an emotional problem (such as feeling depressed or anxious)?

	Yes	No
a) Have you reduced the amount of time you devote to your work or other activities?	1	2
b) Did you do fewer tasks than you would have liked?	1	2
c) You didn't carry out or do any of the activities as carefully as you usually do.	1	2

6- During the last 4 weeks, how have your physical health or emotional problems interfered with your normal social activities, with family, friends or in groups?

Not at all	Slightly	Moderately	Quite a lot	Extremely
1	2	3	4	5

7- How much body pain have you experienced in the last 4 weeks?

None	Very light	Lightweight	Moderate	Grave	A lot
1	2	3	4	5	6

8- During the last 4 weeks, how much has the pain interfered with your normal work (including work inside the home)?

Not at all	A little	Moderately	Quite a lot	Extremely
1	2	3	4	5

9- These questions are about how you feel and how everything has been going for you over the last 4 weeks. For each question, please mark an answer that most closely matches the way you feel about the last 4 weeks.

	All the time	Most of the time	A good part of the time	Some of the time	A small part of the time	Never
a) how long time you have if feeling full of vigor, will, strength?	1	2	3	4	5	6
b) How long have you been feeling very nervous?	1	2	3	4	5	6
c) How long have you been so depressed that nothing can cheer you up?	1	2	3	4	5	6
d) How long have you felt calm or peaceful?	1	2	3	4	5	6
e) How long have you felt energized?	1	2	3	4	5	6
f) How long have you felt discouraged or down?	1	2	3	4	5	6
g) How long have you felt exhausted?	1	2	3	4	5	6
h) How long have you felt like a happy person?	1	2	3	4	5	6
i) How long have you been feeling tired?	1	2	3	4	5	6

10- During the last 4 weeks, how much of your time did your physical health or emotional problems interfere with your social activities (such as visiting friends, relatives, etc.)?

All the time	Most of the time	Some of the time	A small part of the	No part of the time
1	2	3	4	5

11- How true or false is each of the statements for you?

	Definitely true	Most of the time true	I don't know	Most of the time false	Definitely false
a) I tend to get sick a bit more easily than	1	2	3	4	5
b) I'm as healthy as any person who I know	1	2	3	4	5
c) I think my health will get worse	1	2	3	4	5
d) My health is excellent	1	2	3	4	5

SCORE:/100

Signature of researcher: Date: /__/

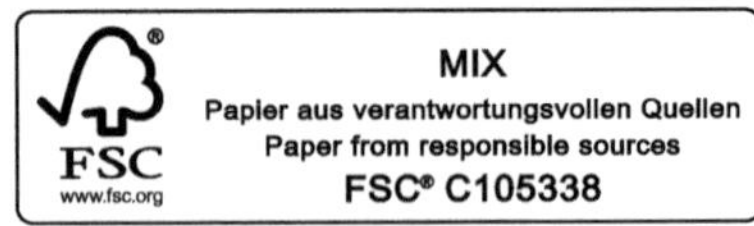

Printed by Books on Demand GmbH, Norderstedt / Germany